Praise for authors' prev

Japanese Women Don't G

'Excellent! A diet that's anti-ageing, slimming and fills you ~~ ~
we sign up?'
Grazia

'A delicious way to stay healthy.'
The Washington Post

'If you need inspiration to change your diet, spending a couple of hours
with Naomi Moriyama should do the trick. She has a slight (but not too
skinny) frame, perfect skin, lots of energy and gleaming hair. She looks 20
years younger than her real age of 45 . . . In short, Japanese people,
especially women, are the healthiest in the world.'
Daily Telegraph

'Incredibly informative and easy to read, full of handy hints . . . the perfect
tool to help you incorporate aspects of the Tokyo kitchen into your diet
and lifestyle, for a slimmer, more energetic and youthful you.'
Health and Fitness Magazine

'The key to Naomi's diet success is the Japanese Country Power Breakfast,
a miso soup chock-full of tofu, vegetables and a whole egg. And there's
truth in her boast: Japanese women have the world's lowest obesity rate
(2.9 per cent to France's 11 per cent) and highest life expectancy (85
years).'
GQ

'The book has plenty of tempting recipes to try and is written in a homely,
anecdotal manner that makes it almost more like a novel than an
instruction guide.'
Daily Star

'The secret is eating plentifully but healthily. Moriyama dishes up tasty
recipes, along with portions of memoir that capture her childhood in
Tokyo.'
You Magazine

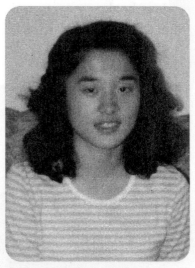

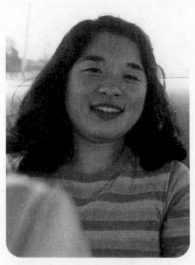

Before: Naomi's first week in America, fresh off the plane from Tokyo, having been raised on a Japanese diet.

After: 8 weeks later Naomi gained 25 pounds after eating a Western-style diet.

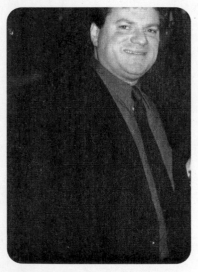

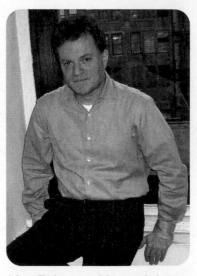

Before: William lands in Tokyo with a 42-inch waist and a pot belly. He was clinically obese.

After: Today, over 30 pounds less, with a 35-inch waist, after adopting a lifestyle of Japanese-style eating.

THE JAPAN DIET

 The secret to effective and lasting weight loss

Naomi Moriyama and William Doyle

with a Foreword by Dr Mabel Blades, Registered Dietitian

Vermilion
LONDON

To our families, especially Chizuko, Shigeo, Marilou and Bill

3 5 7 9 10 8 6 4

First published in the United Kingdom in 2007 by Vermilion,
an imprint of Ebury Publishing
A Random House Group Company

Addresses for companies within
The Random House Group Limited can be found at:
www.randomhouse.co.uk/offices.htm

The Random House Group Limited Reg. No. 954009

A CIP catalogue record for this book
is available from the British Library

ISBN: 9780091917043

The Random House Group Limited supports The Forest Stewardship Council (FSC), the leading international forest certification organisation. All our titles that are printed on Greenpeace approved FSC certified paper carry the FSC logo. Our paper procurement policy can be found at:
www.randomhouse.co.uk/environment

Printed and bound in Great Britain by
CPI Antony Rowe, Chippenham, Wiltshire

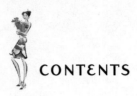

CONTENTS

Acknowledgements		vii
A Note from Naomi: How to Use This Book		viii
Foreword		ix
DAY 1:	Step Into a Dieter's Dream	1
DAY 2:	Come with Me to Tokyo	6
DAY 3:	Understand Why Fad Diets Aren't Working	14
DAY 4:	Open the Holy Grail of Diets	20
DAY 5:	The Foundations of The Japan Diet	24
DAY 6:	How the Japanese Diet Compares with the UK Diet	29
DAY 7:	Open Your Mind to the Japan Diet Attitude	32
DAY 8:	Reach for Realistic, Attainable Goals	37
DAY 9:	Step into a Beautiful World – Right Around the Corner	45
DAY 10:	See the Beauty of Mindful Eating	50
DAY 11:	Liberate Your Dishes and Humanise Your Portions	57

DAY 12: Colour Your Life with Fruit and Vegetables 64

DAY 13: Have a Japan-Style Vegetable Moment 73

DAY 14: Swim in the Good Fats – with Fish 78

DAY 15: Try Some Soya 85

DAY 16: Unleash the Power of Rice and Wholegrains 91

DAY 17: Be Gentle to Your Food 99

DAY 18: Lighten Up Your Beverages 105

DAY 19: The Japan Diet Shopping Guide 113

DAY 20: Jumpstart with Breakfast 119

DAY 21: Integrate Your Exercise 123

DAY 22: The Portable Japan Diet 131

DAYS 23–29: A Japan Diet-Inspired 7-Day Sample Healthy

Eating Plan 137

Day 30: The Days of Magical Eating . . . and an

Eternal Love Affair with Food 152

Sample Japan Diet Meals Based on Recipes 161

The Japan Diet Recipes 166

Tokyo Kitchen Key Ingredients 217

Tokyo Kitchen Utensils 232

Resources 233

Source Notes 243

Index 251

ACKNOWLEDGEMENTS

We thank Clare Hulton, Julia Kellaway, Imogen Fortes, Sarah Bennie, Judy Jamieson-Green and Philippa Collinge of Random House; and Mel Berger, Shana Kelly, Raffaella De Angelis, Tracy Fisher, Evan Goldfried, Jules Lantin, Pat Polite and Merrill Mladineo of William Morris. A special thanks to Frankie Phillips for her analysis and research for our 7-Day Healthy Eating Plan and to Mabel Blades for writing the Foreword and reviewing our book.

We also thank the doctors, scientists, academicians, dietitians and others around the world who contributed their help, ideas, opinions and research to this book, especially: Wayne Furman, William Dietz, Barbara Rolls, David Ludwig, Robert Eckel, Frank Hu, Lawrence Appel, Lewis Kuller, Chizuru Nishida, Toshiie Sakata, Yukio Yamori, Yuji Matsuzawa, Jason Williams, Julia Laflin, Qi Dai, Raj Padwal, Matthew Clarke, Richard Tester, Roger Clemens, Sarah Kennedy, David Keldie, Jane Kirby, Akira Sekikawa, Don Staniford, Joanna Price, Leonard Marks, David Jacobs, Arya Sharma, Jane Teas, Simon Tokumine, Christine Skibola, Lorna Dolci, Charlotte Pinder, Mark Ashen, Steve Hawks, Helen Croker, John Michael Lean, Michikazu Sekine, Jeremy Ferguson, Paul Habojan, Fujio Kayama, Susan Roberts, Claire MacEvilly, Gary Wittert, Ken Hughes, Karol Sikora, David Carpenter, Laura Fleming, Henry Blackburn, Robert Vogel, Ed Yong, Marie Françoise Cachera, Christopher Gardner, Mark Wahlqvist, Tim Fitzgerald, Ann Yelmokas McDermott, France Bellisle, Marly Augusto Cardoso, George Grimble, Ian Caterson, Theresa Nicklas, Benjamin Caballero, Susan Jebb, Alexander Leaf, David Colquhoun, Luigi Fontana, Louise Lambert-Lagacé, Denise Simons-Morton, Gary Ko, Mark Tremblay, Alan Lopez, Diane Wreford, Barbara Isman, Masashi Tanaka, Mary Hind, Shiko Nakamura, Miki, Kazuma, Kasumi and Ayaka Wako, Kate and Joe Hooper and Tsune Moriyama.

A NOTE FROM NAOMI: HOW TO USE THIS BOOK

I am so thrilled that you picked up this book!

The Japan Diet is a 30-day journey of insights, small steps, shortcuts and tips to help you achieve a slimmer you over the long term – by acquiring a lifetime of healthy eating and lifestyle habits.

I designed it to be read, sampled and practised over the course of 30 days and lived for the rest of your life.

I suggest you read it a day at a time, taking time to go through the exercises and reflect on the different points and various new lines of thinking. Think of it as a workbook, something you should write all over, underline, highlight, bookmark and earmark.

I'll take you through The Japan Diet gradually, step by step.

In Weeks 1–3, I'll show you the basics of The Japan Diet and the best lessons of healthy eating and how to put them into action in your life.

In Week 4, I'll show you how to enjoy a sample Healthy Eating Plan inspired by the foundations of The Japan Diet. It is built entirely on takeaway and high-convenience foods you can grab at a sushi takeaway or your local supermarket.

In other words, you don't have to learn how to cook authentic Japanese food to enjoy the benefits of The Japan Diet!

Finally, for the weeks and months ahead, I'll give you a collection of sample meals and delicious, authentic, yet simple and easy, Japanese recipes you can have fun with as you begin exploring The Japan Diet in your life a little deeper.

As we say in Japan, *dozo, meshiagare!* Or, please, enjoy!

Naomi

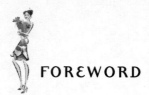

FOREWORD

'Health is one of the most important things in life. Without it, life is not worth living. Without it, you can't enjoy life. Eat delicious healthy foods, otherwise you won't be able to accomplish anything.'

This quote in the book is so true, and with overweight and obesity, as well as the related health problems, being so common in the UK it is so good to see that the authors of *The Japan Diet* do not advocate any 'quick-fix' solution which results in a rapid weight loss followed by an even more rapid weight gain

Instead, they take the reader through 30 days of good, sound advice, which allows a change to a more healthy way of eating. This pattern is reflective of the Japanese way of life with the emphasis on quality and carefully prepared foods, which are slowly enjoyed and not rushed. This is a way of eating in Japan, which results in the population having one of the lowest rates of obesity and coronary heart disease in the world.

To assist the reader there are charts that allow you to reflect on your diet over a period of time as you work towards your goal of weight loss. The 30-day plan introduces Japanese-style eating gradually and also allows the reader to still include the well-liked foods that they normally enjoy while trying new dishes and food experiences.

The Japanese foods suggested in this book are tasty and exquisitely prepared and therefore should appeal to those readers who tend to overeat a more bland diet, based on fast and convenience foods, as the Japanese dishes provide a satisfying taste experience.

Throughout there are quotes from various experts in nutrition to add extra depth to the diet and the emphasis is on good, flavoursome food and recipes.

The advice in *The Japan Diet* also encompasses much of the advice that is generally provided by expert bodies. The authors do recognise that the diet in Japan can be high in salt and recommend ways of reducing this for the reader. Therefore much of the advice will fit in with even therapeutic diets, such as those for diabetes and raised cholesterol levels.

There are lovely snippets of insights into the authors' way of life in Japan and family food preparation, cooking and eating there. The recipes are tempting and easy to follow, but also extremely attractive, and there is a section on information on the ingredients. Therefore even those who cannot easily obtain all of the ingredients locally can make substitutions using more familiar produce.

So, to end with another quote from the book which is extremely pertinent, 'food should be eaten with the eyes as well as the mouth'.

Dr Mabel Blades, PhD, BSc, RD
Dr Blades is a dietitian and nutritionist and an expert in the treatment of disorders by diet. Her work includes food consultancy, recipe development and teaching as well as research and lecturing.

DAY 1

STEP INTO A DIETER'S DREAM

Learn all the rules, then forget them.

- THE POET BASHO

The Japanese people today are living longer and healthier than any other nation on earth.

And they have the lowest rates of obesity in the developed world.

One of the reasons for this is what Japanese people eat – and how they eat it.

It is a diet that is delicious, energising and deeply satisfying.

This book is the story of a pattern of food and lifestyle insights that experts believe can hold the keys to healthy, long-term weight loss – a pattern that I call 'The Japan Diet'.

And it is the story of how you can put these insights into action – easily.

What is The Japan Diet?

The Japan Diet is an attitude and a style of healthy lifetime eating.

It is a celebration of fish, vegetables, rice, soya, fruit and other healthy foods, all gently prepared without heavy sauces or creams and served in modest but filling portions. Its goal is for you to enjoy more satisfaction from fewer calories, more 'good fats' and 'good carbohydrates', less salt, less added sugar and less 'bad fats' and to enjoy regular physical activity.

You can boil The Japan Diet down to twelve basic insights, all of which you can instantly start applying to your everyday food life:

THE JAPAN DIET IN A CAPSULE
12 Steps to Easily Japan-Style Your Life

1. Eat more fish, especially oily fish like salmon, sardines, mackerel and herring.
2. Eat lots more fruit and vegetables, in a rich variety of many types and colours.
3. Japan-style your portions: enjoy moderate helpings on smaller plates.
4. Eat mindfully – relax and eat at a leisurely pace; aim for variety, moderation and balance.
5. Choose foods with less saturated fat, salt, added sugars, and little or no trans fat.
6. Be gentle to your food: cook with heart-healthy oils, such as rapeseed, and healthy techniques, such as steaming.
7. Eat more wholegrain foods like brown rice, wholegrain breads and cereals.
8. Lighten up your beverages: drink fewer sweetened-fizzy drinks and go for unsweetened tea, water and low-fat milk.
9. Think of generous amounts of veggies more often as the star of your meal.
10. Don't skip meals, including breakfast.
11. Get physically active and stay active regularly: moderate exercise, like walking, counts.
12. Think of food as a source of joy, indulgence, good health, positive energy, laughter and celebration. Don't go on a diet. Instead, phase healthy eating habits into your daily diet over the long-term.

Bonus step when you'd like to try Japanese foods: sample some Japan-style foods at your supermarket, takeaway or Japanese speciality shop, such as edamame soya beans, green tea, tofu, sushi and sea vegetables; and try some of the recipes at the back of this book.

The *premise* of The Japan Diet is that there are some beautiful lessons you can learn from the best of traditional Japanese food habits and that they are very easy to put into action in your own life.

The *philosophy* of The Japan Diet is gradual weight loss and long-term weight maintenance through healthy eating, active lifestyle and the best expert advice – with a Japan-style twist.

The ideas in this book are inspired by my personal story of growing up in Japan, getting fat on the American diet and then losing all the extra fat and keeping it off after rediscovering the art and beauty of the Japanese diet.

Many of these ideas are supported by a cross-section of the latest expert recommendations on good nutrition and healthy weight loss today, including the suggestions of the UK Food Standards Agency (FSA), the British Dietetic Association (BDA) and the World Health Organization (WHO).

A distinguished panel of over 50 experts contributed their insights and opinions to this book and its predecessor, *Japanese Women Don't Get Old or Fat,* in a series of in-depth interviews.

They are leading doctors, professors, scientists, dietitians and researchers in the UK, the US, Japan, Europe and Asia and include members of the BDA, the Medical Research Council, the Japanese Society for the Study of Obesity and faculty members at some of the world's leading universities and medical schools. The opinions reached by my co-author William Doyle and me are, of course, entirely our own.

The Japan Diet is *not* a restrictive set of rules.

It is *not* a rigid programme.

It is *not* a crash diet.

It is *not* a programme of denial, semi-starvation, nor of trying to manipulate your body chemistry by eliminating food groups.

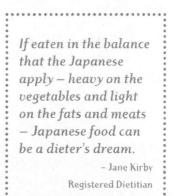

If eaten in the balance that the Japanese apply – heavy on the vegetables and light on the fats and meats – Japanese food can be a dieter's dream.

– Jane Kirby
Registered Dietitian

The Japan Diet is not a miracle diet, nor a magic bullet. I have never tried a fad diet. I never thought I needed to, or wanted to. Even if I tried, I wouldn't last more than a few days. I am not that disciplined, anyway. Following a complicated programme seems so restricting. What do I order when I go out with my friends? Fad diets don't seem natural to me at all.

The Japan Diet is a style of healthy eating based on traditional dietary patterns and habits evolved over thousands of years of Japanese food history and culture, empowered by the latest expert nutritional advice.

You should think of The Japan Diet as a way of working towards the goals of healthy eating suggestions of the most knowledgeable authorities, such as the FSA and the BDA.

Losing weight can be extremely hard and the experts don't always agree on how to do it. Weight gain and obesity are exquisitely complex medical and scientific subjects and new discoveries and research breakthroughs are happening all the time.

Neither this nor any other book has all the answers and there is no guarantee that you will lose weight on this or any other healthy eating approach. This book should be one of many resources you consult on your road to a slimmer you.

The best authority, of course, is yourself, working with the advice of your GP or dietitian and armed with the latest, best nutritional information.

The good news is that many experts are starting to agree on some of the most important foundations of healthy weight loss and these foundations are what The Japan Diet is based on.

The Japan Diet is *not* about eating Japanese food all the time. I don't know many people who do that, even in Japan.

It is about eating *Japan-style*. There's a big difference.

You can get fat on Japanese food, or British food, or Mediterranean food. And you can lose weight on them, too. The key words are 'healthy choices' and 'healthy balance'.

The Japan Diet is a new attitude towards diet and healthy eating that you can customise to your taste and your preferences.

The Japan Diet is what you make it.

My philosophy is that cooking is fun, shopping for food is fun and eating is *really* fun. I believe the purpose of food is good health, positive energy, indulgence, celebration and joy with the people we love.

> *The traditional Japanese diet is among the healthiest in the world. It is rich in vegetables from the land and sea, cooked and raw, fruit, vegetable protein such as tofu and fish. In addition, Japanese culture places an emphasis on quality, rather than quantity, and enjoyment of the meal, rather than just getting full. In this way, a moderate-sized meal can be much more satisfying than a much larger meal, for example fast food.*
>
> – Dr David Ludwig, Director, Obesity Program
> Children's Hospital Boston, Harvard Medical School

Do you remember the last delicious Japanese meal you had?

Maybe it was a tasty sushi lunch, or a steaming bowl of veggies and Japanese noodles, or a mouth-watering Japan-style dinner with little appetisers and fish and rice.

Can you remember how you felt after you ate it?

If you're like me, you didn't feel over-stuffed or sleepy, but satisfied, energised, lean and healthy.

That's the power of Japan-style eating.

If you've never had a traditional Japanese-style meal, don't worry. I will take you there in the pages of this book.

You can start feeling this way every day, by applying the lessons of The Japan Diet to your super-busy life.

Together, let's fall in love with food again . . . in a whole new way.

As you go to sleep tonight, dream of delicious days we will soon be having together, in a land that is on the other side of the world and just around the corner.

DAY 2

COME WITH ME TO TOKYO

Let's go across the sea for a taste of the Japan Diet

I got fat in America.

I grew up in Japan and was raised on the traditional Japanese food and 'Japanised' Western food cooked by my mother Chizuko in her Tokyo kitchen. In the summer, I ate Japanese country-style cooking at my grandmother Tsune's farm in the mountains of Mie Prefecture.

Then, when I went to college in the United States, I gained 11 kg (25 lbs) in just two months.

I gained all that weight by eating a typical Western diet of big portions of meatloaf, mashed potatoes drenched in delicious thick brown gravy, cheeseburgers, pasta, pizza, chips, cakes and pies, piles of pancakes swimming in melted butter and syrup, giant boats of banana splits and chocolate chip cookies in large quantities. The relatively few vegetables I ate were often overcooked and lathered in butter or creamy salad dressing.

Sounds kind of great, doesn't it?

For the next two years, all I had was this typical American fare. And I will confess to you – after I had got used to it, I loved every bite of American food.

But the food really made me chubby. This was rural Illinois, where the car culture and long winters combined practically to eliminate walking from the average person's lifestyle.

I totally exploded. I burst out of my clothes! I tried to exercise the extra 11 kg away, but I couldn't shake it off. The entire food culture seemed geared to making me overeat, to the point where I thought it was normal after every meal to feel so stuffed that I wanted to unbuckle my trousers and lie down on the floor.

My clothes got tighter and tighter and then I couldn't fit into them. I tried to put on a pink linen skirt, but was amazed to realise that the hooks on the waistline had about a 7-cm (3-in) gap and a deep inhale wasn't going to close it. None of my skirts and trousers fitted me any more and they sat in a box in my wardrobe for almost two years.

What does it feel like to be fat?

In my case, the extra weight made me feel lazy, tired and sweaty. I didn't want to move or walk around as much. It was a vicious circle. It forced me into a wide range of inconveniences. I had less energy, sometimes even shortness of breath. It was pretty exhausting.

Then I went back to live with my parents in Tokyo.

Within weeks of eating 'Japan-style' at my mother Chizuko's Tokyo kitchen, I was losing all the extra weight, without any real effort, simply by switching to my mother's Japanese home cooking, supported by the walking-intense Tokyo lifestyle. I lost the weight at a rate of ½ to 1 kg (1 to 2 lb) a week, which is exactly the pace, I later found out, that is recommended by medical experts.

I was not even trying to lose it. It just happened. Soon, I was back to my old weight again.

I can remember what it first felt like . . .

What Westerners can learn from Japanese food and their food habits is that Japanese food opens a new series of possibilities in tasty, healthy eating.
– Dr David Colquhoun, Consultant Cardiologist
Associate Professor of Medicine, The University of Queensland

It is morning in Japan. The sun is up on a warm early summer day.

'*Ohayo!* (Good morning!),' I call out to my family, not anyone in particular, as I walk into the combination living–dining room of my parents' apartment.

I sit down for breakfast at the dining table, all dressed up to go to work at my new job at Tokyo Disneyland, which is still under construction. I am an English language translator for the legendary costume designer Jack Muhs from the original California Disneyland, and my job involves following him with a notepad and pen around the emerging Magic Kingdom and Cinderella Castle, in my hard hat and big construction boots, then reviewing costumes on stage with Mickey and Minnie Mouse.

The 7am news is running on TV, but I am not really watching it. Japanese phrases sound a bit weird, since I've not watched Japanese TV in two years.

On the table, my mother Chizuko has already spread out plates, utensils and a partial breakfast. I don't think the idea of skipping breakfast has ever once crossed her mind her whole life. She is in her compact kitchen juggling a few items, as usual.

A typical breakfast at my parents is 'Japanised-Western', ever since I was a little girl. Coffee is freshly brewed in a pot. I like my coffee black. I take a sip, it hits a certain point at the back of my brain and feels good. A couple of pieces of thick toast sit in a basket in the middle of the table, still warm from the toaster oven. They are crispy on the outside and fluffy inside.

Around the time I was going to high school, our family somehow collectively agreed that thick toast tastes better than thin toast. I take a half slice, break the edge off and toss it into my mouth.

Chizuko comes out of the kitchen, which is not even one metre from where I'm sitting, with a familiar well-worn frying pan in her left hand and a spatula in her right. She scoops sautéed shredded cabbage topped with an egg, sunny-side up, and places it on a medium-size plate in front of my father, who sits on the other side of the table. She says to him, 'Please start while it's hot.'

With the spatula, she scoops another mound of cabbage topped with an egg from the pan and slides it onto my plate. Hot steam rises out of the mound. I smell the sweetness of the cabbage and the specks of freshly cracked black pepper all over the egg. While my mother walks around the table to serve my younger sister Miki, who is in her high school uniform, I swing into the kitchen and grab a bottle of Worcestershire sauce from the fridge. The sauce's spicy sweet flavour blends perfectly with the egg-cabbage dish. I take a bite and say, 'Oisheee!', or 'Delicious – tastes great!'

I look up from my breakfast and glance at the upper corner of the TV screen now and then to check the official time, so as not to miss my train. I have small casual chats with my father, mostly about what I am up to at work today.

Chizuko brings out small bowls of clear soup with green leafy vegetables. She makes pa-ta pa-ta sounds with her slippers (we don't wear shoes in the house) and sits down to join us.

My dad pours her some coffee. She nods to him, 'Ah, thank you.' She takes her coffee black too.

I glance at the time on the TV screen again. It's time to go.

I stand up and announce the customary, 'Gochiso-sama!' which means 'That was a feast!' My mother says, 'Are you already finished?' She offers me more toast, a typical Chizuko move. 'No, Mum, I've had enough, I've got to get to work!'

At 6.30 that evening I come home. I am starving.

Japanese short-grain rice is steaming in the rice cooker.

As usual, my mum is orchestrating several dishes. On a typical night it will be a miso soup, two or three vegetable-based dishes, a fish or small meat dish, often cooked with other veggies, plus a bowl or two of fluffy, slightly sticky rice. Dessert will be sliced fruit and green tea.

I tuck into dinner and soon I'm feeling warm and fluffy myself.

The food is absolutely delicious and totally filling and, just like the American food I had become addicted to, I am loving every bite, but in a distinctly different way.

● ● ● ● ●

After a few weeks of this healthy eating rhythm, of regular nutritious meals, lots of veggies, city walking and very little junk food, I was becoming my real self again.

I felt lean and energetic. And I felt fantastic! My clothes were getting looser.

I was delighted to feel my old clothes were fitting me again. I felt all my extra kilos melting away. And soon they were all gone. I was back to less than 48 kg (7 st 7 lb) which, for my small stature (155 cm/5 ft 2 in), is considered a normal body mass index (BMI). This is a figure obtained by dividing your weight in kilograms (kg) by your height in metres (m) squared. A BMI of over 25 is defined as overweight and over 30 is defined as obese. You can check yours online by searching for a BMI calculator, for example at the British Dietetic Association Weight Wise website: www.bdaweightwise.com/lose/lose_bmi.aspx

After I moved to New York, years later, when my husband and co-author Billy and I first visited my mother's Tokyo kitchen together, he fell totally in love with her food. He loved it so much that we started re-creating it at our home in New York.

We applied many of the super-easy lessons we observed at her table in our home, too: regular meals, not skipping breakfast, often basing meals around fish, veggies and fruit, a small bowl or two of short-grain rice with every meal. Taking time to savour every little bite.

We were amazed to discover that in the process of eating regular healthy Japan-style meals every day, Billy started losing a good deal of weight over time and feeling great. He was eating this way because he liked the taste of the food, not to lose weight.

Exercising was becoming easier for him. His trousers were getting too big for him. He used to be a big fellow with an 'extra large' shirt size, but eventually he was down to 'large' and sometimes nearly fitting into a 'medium'. He was pleasantly surprised, as was I.

He gradually went from a 105-cm (42-in) waist down to 87 cm (35 in); from over 100 kg (15 stone 10 lb), or technically 'obese' for his height (a BMI of over 30), down to a healthy 'normal' BMI of around 84 kg (13 stone 3 lb), where he's stayed for years and remains today.

I think of Tokyo as 'The Infinite Gourmet City', a place of almost limitless size and an endless horizon of food choices and food temptations. There is more magnificently good food in Tokyo than most other places on Earth. But Japan has also become a victim of the low-nutrition, high-calorie food industry invasion. There is every chocolatey, gooey, super-sweetened food temptation you could imagine, as well as some thoroughly awful deep-fried, over-processed, fatty-and-salty fast food and junk food.

In that sense, I think no matter where you go in the developed world, our daily lives are a constant challenge as we navigate through the infinite array of food choices that bombard us every day. Around every corner there is a dietary treasure or a dietary disaster.

We didn't realise it at the time, but my mother had been feeding us her version of The Japan Diet, our phrase for a traditional style of healthy eating, that we later found out is considered to be close to an international gold standard of healthy eating by leading experts around the world.

Like many mothers and grandmothers in the Far East, the UK and the Mediterranean, my mother has somehow stayed connected to a highly nutritious, traditional healthy diet. It is an organic process that she follows, not because it's on the cutting edge of nutritional science, but because it naturally feels like the right thing to do. The wisdom had been passed down to her from her parents, Hamako and Kiyoshi, and their parents and ancestors going all the way back in time.

At almost the exact moment in history that I returned to Tokyo after college, the Japanese nation was enjoying a fleeting Golden Age of Nutritional Balance. The government of Japan now considers the year 1980 as the point in time when the national diet was in a state of 'nutritional balance' of Eastern and Western food styles and calorie content, and with a healthy balance of food types eaten.

While you might say that the weight loss Billy and I experienced was a happy accident, we've lived with this approach for years now and we can tell you it has transformed our lives in a very positive way. In these pages, we will deconstruct the Japanese diet for you, show you its healthiest lessons and how to incorporate them into your own life.

Since we are neither medical nor scientific experts, we sought out some of the world's top experts on diet and nutrition to try to understand what we experienced.

We asked them for their opinions on weight loss, long-term weight maintenance, healthy and unhealthy eating, and how the Japanese diet compares with the typical Western diet, which unfortunately represents a negative pattern towards which many people around the world are shifting, even in Japan.

In discussing these subjects, the experts were passionate, excited, enthusiastic, curious, sometimes sceptical and very candid as they debated their opinions and speculations.

And they have some fascinating things to tell us.

Dr William Dietz is Director of Division of Nutrition and Physical Activity for the US Centers for Disease Control and a leading expert on global health and obesity issues. He recalled:

I lived in Japan for three years as a child. When I revisited Japan as an adult, I had some wonderful experiences with Japanese food and Japanese-style eating and the types of foods that were served and how they were served.

I have this quite distinctive memory of being in a restaurant and served an appetiser with a beautiful sugar maple leaf that was changing colour, just to decorate the plate.

In addition to the quality of the food and fish and the omega-3 fatty acids and vegetables and soya and the absence of trans fats, one of the things that is most notable about Japanese eating and Japanese cooking is that there's a lot of emphasis on style and presentation, and an emphasis on small portions, so the quantity of food is counterbalanced by the style in which it's presented.

The eating experience is not driven by quantity; it's driven by taste and style.

I traveled to a very rustic town in northern Japan and joined in a banquet with a family of rice farmers. There were about 10 of us seated around a table with a pot of boiling water and stock in the center in which we cooked seafood. What was striking was the seafood was so diverse – there must have been 10 different types of seafood and it was all served with a minimum of extras. So the emphasis was on the food, not the condiments in which the food was dipped or prepared.

That meal was notable for its simplicity and the lack of externality. It tasted great.

The feeling I have when I eat Japanese food is that I feel full but not overstuffed. The food doesn't seem as heavy, perhaps because the fat content is so much lower. If you look at sushi or sashimi, they are filling foods, but they don't have a very high fat content. They're principally protein and carbohydrates. Soya is a pretty healthful product and it picks up the flavours of whatever else you're preparing and cooking it with.

In Japan, a typical breakfast can include a lot of vegetables, which is quite a contrast from what you get in any other country I've visited.

The Japanese are also seeing an increase in obesity. They're quite concerned about it because Asians tend to develop the complications of obesity at lower Body Mass Indices than Western populations. What's driving the obesity epidemic in Japan is no clearer there than it is here, but there are concerns about the Westernization of the food supply, and inactivity – the same concerns that have been raised in the West.

UNDERSTAND WHY FAD DIETS AREN'T WORKING

The bad news is that fad diets don't work.

It is becoming painfully clear.

We are getting bigger than ever.

If you're feeling rather heavy these days, you're not alone.

We have dieted, detoxed, carb-counted, cleansed, re-balanced, irrigated, meal-skipped, food-restricted, food-timed, food-combined, fasted, protein-shaked, fat-burned, obsessed and denied ourselves to the point where we now weigh more than we ever did.

Despite millions of diet books sold and billions of pounds spent fighting fat, so many people are putting on so much weight so quickly that in October 2005 the new chairwoman of the UK's Food Standards Agency, Dame Deirdre Hutton, told *The Times*, 'When you look at the number of people medically affected by poor diet in terms of ill health or early death from a diet-related disease, we have to do something about it. If you look at the level of obesity in kids and the way it is growing, it's terrifying.'

Over 30,000 premature deaths in the UK are blamed on obesity. Levels of obesity have tripled in England since 1980. Using the international definition of obesity, the International Obesity Task Force estimates that 22 per cent of adults in England are obese, 20 per cent in Scotland and 18 per cent in Wales; versus a whopping 32 per cent in the USA – and a tiny 3 per cent in Japan, the lowest rate of all the developed nations. Children in the UK are being diagnosed with formerly 'adult' illnesses such as Type 2 diabetes, hypertension and cardiovascular diseases. Shadow Health Secretary Andrew Lansley said, 'In the last decade British children have got fatter faster than anywhere else in Western Europe.'

The obesity problem is a world-wide crisis and a public health time-bomb.

It is spreading into the historically lean regions of the Mediterranean and Asia, including Italy, Spain, India and China. An obesity crisis has even erupted in the healthiest and leanest nation in the developed world – Japan, although it is still five to 10 years behind the United States.

Things are getting so bad in the USA that last year the Surgeon General, Richard Carmona, called obesity 'the terror within' and said that unless we do something about it 'the magnitude of the dilemma will dwarf 9–11 or any other terrorist attempt'. Dr Meir Stampfer of the Harvard School of Public Health told *WebMD News*: 'It is just staggering. This whole epidemic of obesity is sweeping across the country. One of the difficulties is it's becoming the norm to be overweight. People look down at their bellies, see other people's bellies and see they are average. But in this country, if you are average, you are way overweight.'

I'm not talking about being a little overweight, or having a few extra pounds. Personally, I hate the way our culture can often demonise and ridicule overweight people and how it can obsess over thinness. And I think it's beautiful that the media is finally starting to portray women in more realistic sizes and shapes.

What worries me is obesity, which is usually defined as a body mass index of over 30. Obesity isn't just an inconvenience or a cosmetic issue: it can make you very sick. It is literally a killer disease. According to the World Health Organization, obesity raises your risk of Type 2 diabetes, cardiovascular disease, hypertension and stroke, respiratory disease, osteoarthritis, problems with pregnancy, gallbladder disease and certain forms of cancer.

The obesity problem is almost out of control and the world is getting fatter and fatter. How can this be happening – when we seem to be drowning in a sea of fad diets, diet pills, celebrity diet crazes, fitness gurus and health information?

Why are we getting so fat?

The problem it seems, is due to an increasingly extreme imbalance in the quality and quantity of the food we eat and the way that imbalance interacts with our lifestyle.

According to Dame Dierdre, of the FSA, overall, 'We are eating too much saturated fat, too much salt and too much sugar and not enough fruit and vegetables and starchy carbohydrates.'

In addition, according to the theories of experts who have studied the problem of obesity, we are:

- Eating more calories than we burn off, or falling into a 'calorie surfeit'.
- Not exercising enough.
- Becoming more sedentary in our daily lives, for example, watching more TV and spending leisure time using computers instead of being physically active.
- Eating more super-size fast-food meals.
- Eating portion sizes that have exploded in size over the past decades.
- Eating more junk food and snacks.
- Eating more unhealthy takeaway and ready meals.
- Eating more animal fat, hydrogenated fats and trans fats.
- Eating fewer complex carbohydrates and dietary fibre.
- Eating more processed food.
- Being exposed to the wrong nutritional choices at our schools and offices.
- Drinking too many sweetened fizzy drinks.
- Eating food that is more 'calorie dense' and 'nutrient poor'.
- Losing the skills, time or desire to make healthier meals for ourselves and our families.

By the way, this pattern completely matches my fat years in America.

So many people are going on and off fad diets that don't work. Most 'diets', as currently defined, simply don't work over the long term. A fad diet may temporarily result in weight loss simply by reducing your daily calorie intake, but as soon as you 'go off' the diet you can swiftly regain what you lost, plus even more weight.

A rising chorus of experts has even been blasting the very idea of 'dieting'.

Dr Frankie Phillips, spokesperson for the British Dietetic Association, explained that: 'The main misconception is that dieting is a quick-fix solution to what is, in essence, a long-term maintenance problem, which people need to get to grips with if they are to achieve a healthy weight in the long term.'

In general, explains Dr Robert Eckel, President of the American Heart Association and Professor of Medicine at the University of Colorado, 'Most crash diets end up crashing. People do lose a lot of weight fairly quickly but they bounce back within a period of months. We're really concerned about the quick fix mentality.' His suggestion is to modestly reduce your daily calories over time through healthy eating combined with exercise, expecting about a pound or two of weight loss per week.

Despite testimonial ads, anecdotes and word-of-mouth rave reviews, you will find an amazingly small amount of real research on which, if any, popular diets actually work over the long term.

In the meantime, we are bombarded with bad diet advice from dubious experts.

We are swamped with news bites from researchers who sometimes jump to global conclusions based on small studies of nervous laboratory rats. When Drs Lisa Schwartz and Steven Woloshin, of Dartmouth Medical School, USA, analysed press releases about scientific studies, they found that they often omit basic facts about the studies and fail to highlight important limitations.

I think that screenwriter William Goldman's famous quip about Hollywood, 'nobody knows anything', should apply to the diet field as well. 'The reality is we don't yet know a good way to prevent obesity,' said Dr Susan Yanovski MD, director of the obesity and eating disorders programme at the US National Institute of Diabetes and Digestive and Kidney Diseases. 'We are in our infancy in terms of understanding this disorder.'

As soon as a diet trend such as Atkins or the glycaemic index takes hold, well-credentialled authorities emerge to attack it.

Look at the 'low carb' debate of recent years, for example. Critics jumped all over the Atkins Diet, then the Atkins parent company went bankrupt in 2005 and today there is lingering mass public confusion over carbohydrates. 'It's amazing how few good studies have looked at how different carbohydrates affect weight loss,' observed highly respected nutrition researcher Dr Walter Willett, chair of the nutrition department at the Harvard School of Public Health. He described the long-term evidence on weight loss as 'meagre'.

However, long-term randomised trials of different diets on human beings, the hypothetical 'gold standard' in such research, are rarely even attempted, since it's nearly impossible to get people to adhere to a specific diet for five, 10 or 20 years.

Assistant Professor Christopher Gardner, of the University of Stanford School of Medicine, told us, for example, 'What we should do is randomly assign 100,000 people to eat a lot of soya, or not, and follow them for 100 years and see who lives longer. And that's never going to happen.' So what we're stuck with, said Gardner, are imperfect studies with significant limitations. 'You'll never get the perfect studies,' he concluded, 'so what you do is piece together the different parts of the puzzle.'

Part of the problem with diets is that nutritional research often focuses on one or two isolated nutrients or foods only, not overall eating patterns.

'Many studies have looked at dietary fats, cholesterol, carbohydrates, minerals and vitamins, but most of these study minerals or compounds in isolation,' explained Dr Frank Hu, assistant professor of nutrition at the Harvard School of Public Health. 'But in reality,' he reported, 'people eat complex meals rather than isolated nutrients. In those meals there are thousands of minerals and compounds that may have synergistic [working together] or antagonistic [counteracting each other] effects.'

There is also the near-impossibility of disentangling and measuring all the many factors that can impact on people's weight and health, including food combinations, lifestyle, genetics, attitude, exercise and spiritual well-being. 'Nothing is ever as straightforward as it seems when you are talking about diet,' noted Professor Karol Sikora, professor of cancer medicine at the Imperial College School of Medicine.

Diet and nutrition may be an almost infinitely complex puzzle.

Then what are we left to do?

Let's start by opening our eyes to something beautiful that's happening . . .

DAY 4

OPEN THE HOLY GRAIL OF DIETS

In the distance, the fog is lifting.
The sun is starting to sparkle through the trees.
And we are beginning to see the vision of A Holy Grail of
    Healthy Diets.
What's inside is beautiful and delicious.

The Good News: A 'Holy Grail of Diets' is beginning to appear.

Inside the Grail, there is a number of healthy eating patterns that many experts agree can be delicious, effective and sustainable ways to achieve and maintain health and a healthy weight over the long term.

They have names like the 'Balance of Good Health' (UK Food Standards Agency), the 'Healthwise Plan' (British Dietetic Association), 'Dietary Approaches to Stop Hypertension' (or 'DASH') diet to lower high blood pressure (US National Institutes of Health), the 'Therapeutic Lifestyle Changes' (or 'TLC') diet to lower cholesterol, 'The Harvard Healthy Eating Plan', 'Weight Watchers' and the 'No Fad Diet' (American Heart Association).

The healthy diets inside the Grail sometimes have different suggestions, such as what percentage of your calories should be from fat as opposed to protein, things like that. But what is striking is how similar the different plans often are, and how many points of consensus are emerging among experts.

What do the experts agree on?

One of the biggest points of agreement is that the key to losing weight over the long term is not to 'go on a diet' but to adopt a healthy eating plan that includes dietary and lifestyle changes that you stick to over time. As Dr John J. Whyte and Dr Robert N. Marting wrote in the medical journal *Patient Care*, people 'need to focus less on dieting and more on healthy eating'.

The FSA, for example, defines a healthy balanced diet as containing 'a variety of types of food, including lots of fruit, vegetables and starchy foods, such as wholemeal bread and wholegrain cereals; some protein-rich foods, such as meat, fish, eggs and lentils; and some dairy foods'. The Agency has boiled it down to what it calls:

> *People who succeed at maintaining a dramatic weight loss have changed their mindset and priorities and have made exercise and healthy eating among the top priorities in their lives.*
>
> – Dr Michael Dansinger
> Obesity Expert
> Tufts-New England Medical Center

Eight Top Tips for Eating Well

1. Base your meals on starchy foods such as bread, cereals, rice, pasta and potatoes – and try to choose wholegrain varieties whenever you can.

2. Eat lots of fruit and vegetables – aim to eat at least five portions a day.

3. Eat more fish – aim for at least two portions of fish a week, including a portion of oily fish.

4. Cut down on saturated fat and sugar.

5. Try to eat less salt – no more than 6 g a day, or no more than 2.5 g of sodium.

6. Get active and try to be a healthy weight.

7. Drink plenty of water – about six to eight glasses (1.2 litres/2 pints) of water or other fluids a day.

8. Don't skip breakfast.

This may seem rather simple, if not boring. It looks like much the same advice our mothers and grandmothers in England, Europe, North America and Asia have been telling us for generations.

But it's looking more and more like they are the basic foundations of the Holy Grail of Healthy Diets.

Many other authorities are endorsing these same kinds of tips. They include groups such as the World Health Organization, the UK Heart Foundation, the British Dietetic Association and the US National Institutes of Health, representing the collective wisdom of literally thousands of scientists, doctors, researchers and dietitians around the world.

In 2003, the World Health Organization published the results of a study by 30 leading experts around the world who reviewed the best available scientific evidence on the connections between diet, nutrition and physical activity – and chronic diseases like obesity. Their findings on the subject of weight, summarised here, are a synthesis of hundreds of medical and scientific studies:

What the Best Scientific Evidence Says:

Strength of Evidence	DECREASES THE RISK of Weight Gain and Obesity	INCREASES THE RISK of Weight Gain and Obesity
Convincing	- Regular physical activity: one hour per day of moderate-intensity activity such as walking on most days of the week needed to maintain a healthy body weight - High intake of dietary fibre from foods like wholegrain cereals, fruits and vegetables	- Sedentary lifestyles - High intake of calorie-dense, nutrient-poor foods like processed foods high in fat and/or sugars
Probable	- Home and school environments that support healthy food choices for children	- Heavy marketing of calorie-dense foods and fast-food outlets - High intake of sugar-sweetened soft drinks and fruit juices
Possible	- Low glycaemic index foods - 'Flexible restraint' eating patterns	- Large portion sizes - High proportion of food prepared outside the home - 'Rigid restraint/periodic loss of inhibition' eating patterns
Insufficient	- Increased eating frequency	- Alcohol

Source: 'Diet, Nutrition and the Prevention of Chronic Diseases', report of WHO/FAO Expert Consultation

Here's another point the experts agree on: calories really count. In fact, they are the basic formula that determines how we lose weight.

The equation for weight loss is amazingly simple – eat fewer calories than you burn off. The US National Institutes of Health puts it this way: 'Your body weight is controlled by the number of calories you eat and the number of calories you use each day. To lose weight you need to take in fewer calories than you use.'

'Energy in – energy out', which is the same thing as 'calories in – calories out'. That's the formula. 'A calorie is a calorie is a calorie,' explained Samantha Heller, a dietitian at the New York University Medical Center. 'You can get fat eating healthy food and you can lose weight eating candy bars. It's just how much energy in the form of food that you take in and how much you put out physically.' The idea is to consume fewer calories than we burn, while taking in foods that make our body healthy.

Finally, many experts agree that we should eat much less so-called 'bad fats' such as saturated fat, trans fats and partially hydrogenated fats.

It turns out that there is a nation that has enjoyed a diet that comes close in many respects to achieving a number of the healthy eating recommendations of the world's top nutritional experts.

It is a country that eats fewer calories, more modest portions, more fish, more vegetable products as a proportion of its diet – and less sugar and less bad fats.

In the process, it has become the leanest nation in the developed world and the nation with the highest healthy longevity on Earth.

It is Japan.

Together, let's explore some of its most interesting lessons.

DAY 5

THE FOUNDATIONS OF THE JAPAN DIET

What, specifically, is the Japanese diet?

Historically, the traditional foundation of the Japanese diet is a celebration of fish, rice, soya and vegetables, all gently prepared without heavy sauces or creams, and served in modest portions on pretty little dishes. As my mother says in her Tokyo kitchen, 'Food should be eaten with the eyes as well as the mouth,' and 'the best cooking is the least cooking.'

Today, many people in Japan adhere to at least part of this philosophy, while many others are shifting to highly Westernised ways of eating – both good and bad.

Traditional Japanese meals are based largely on what I call 'The Seven Pillars of Japanese Home Cooking': fish, vegetables, rice, soya, fruit, noodles and tea. Meat is included in smaller portions than in the West, almost like a garnish.

This style of eating delivers some of the healthiest new trends in dieting – good fats like omega-3s from oily fish, good plant-based carbohydrates, vitamins, minerals and fibre from vegetables, and beautiful portion control. A classic Japanese home-cooked meal is a bowl of soya miso soup, a bowl of fluffy short-grain rice, cooked and eaten without butter or oil (it's that delicious!), and three side dishes such as grilled fish, garnished tofu and vegetables simmered in stock or sautéed in healthy oil such as rapeseed oil.

A dessert is often an assortment of seasonal fruits, peeled, sliced and arranged on a pretty plate. Western desserts such as ice cream and cakes may be offered, but in much smaller portions than in the West. And a cup of Japanese green tea without milk or sugar makes the perfect finish to a meal.

You feel full and satisfied, because the whole meal is enjoyed at a leisurely pace and you can have seconds or even thirds of the modest-size portions, if you wish. Japanese people love Western-style foods as well, such as pasta, burgers and pizza, but 'Japanised' and in smaller portions.

> *Plant-based diets like the Japanese or Asian diets are a combination of high consumption of vegetables, fruits, grain products including rice and also a high consumption of seafood. A dietary pattern higher in fruits, vegetables, wholegrains and fish/sea food has been consistently associated with a lower risk of chronic diseases. These kinds of plant-based foods certainly have had a lot of scientific support in the past several decades in terms of their benefits on cardiovascular disease, cancer prevention and also longevity.*
>
> – Professor Frank Hu
> Harvard University School of Public Health

Why look to Japan for dietary lessons?
Here are four reasons:

- Japanese adults today have the lowest obesity rate in the developed world.
- Japanese women have the longest life expectancy out of all 192 nations on earth – 86 years, according to the World Health Organization's 2006 World Health Report.
- Even better, Japanese women have the most years of healthy life expectancy, enjoying the most years of full health, over 5.5 years more, for example, than women in the UK.

- Japanese men rank top among all the world's males in terms of both total longevity and total years of healthy longevity, despite a shocking 46 per cent smoking rate (compared with the rate of 14 per cent for Japanese women).

A number of experts see parallels between the Japanese diet and diets that they consider to be healthy and sustainable, and links between Japanese eating patterns and good health. They also note some negative aspects to Japanese eating habits: too much sodium, a major constituent of salt (which is why I always suggest lower sodium options), and the fact that the Japanese are eating more junk food. Some experts suggest that the Japanese should eat even more protein and fresh vegetables.

Much has been made of the fact that Japanese people have the highest longevity in the world, but what's even more impressive is the fact that they enjoy *the most years in full health*. As this chart shows, Japanese people today live the longest, healthiest lives:

Projected Number of Years Lived in Full Health

Country	Total Population	Males	Females
Japan	**75.0**	**72.3**	**77.7**
San Marino	73.4	70.9	75.9
Sweden	73.3	71.9	74.8
Switzerland	73.2	71.1	75.3
Monaco	72.9	70.7	75.2
Iceland	72.8	72.1	73.6
Italy	72.2	70.7	74.7
Spain	72.6	69.9	75.3
Australia	72.6	70.9	74.3
Andorra	72.2	69.8	74.3
Canada	72.2	70.1	74.0
France	72.2	69.3	74.7
Norway	72.0	70.4	73.6

Germany	71.8	69.6	74.0
Luxembourg	71.5	69.3	73.7
Israel	71.4	70.5	72.3
Netherlands	71.2	69.7	72.6
Belgium	71.1	68.9	73.3
Finland	71.1	68.7	73.5
Greece	71.0	69.1	72.9
Malta	71.0	69.7	72.3
New Zealand	70.8	69.5	72.2
United Kingdom	70.6	69.1	72.1
Singapore	70.1	68.8	71.3
Denmark	69.8	68.6	71.1
Ireland	69.8	68.1	71.5
Slovenia	69.5	66.6	72.3
United States	69.3	67.2	71.3

Source: WHO World Health Report 2004, survey of all 192 nations. Definition: on average, a newborn today could expect to live so many years in full health if he or she were to experience the current rates of mortality and disability at all ages until they die. The data provide an expectation of their future lifetime spent in full health.

Isn't it all in the genes?

You might think that the Japanese are just naturally healthier. Well, genes can help, but less than you might think.

Several 'migrant studies' of Japanese people who move to Brazil, Hawaii or the mainland United States have shown that when Japanese people change to a more 'Western' diet and lifestyle, they begin to experience diet-related health problems typical of Western societies, suggesting that Japanese genes don't provide a great deal of protection, if any.

For example, Professor Lewis Kuller, MD, of the University of Pittsburgh Graduate School of Public Health, has noticed that Japanese men born around or after World War II have had surprisingly lower rates of coronary heart disease and atherosclerosis compared with the USA.

'The first hypothesis would be that this is just genetic: that they have the right genes and they can eat anything they damn please and they won't get coronary artery disease,' Dr Kuller said. 'But that's not true,' he reports, 'because the Japanese who have migrated to Hawaii or Brazil or the US have quite high rates of disease. That's a one- or two- generation migration, and your genes can't change that fast.'

Overall, the Japanese have done well with their diet, in the sense that their total cancer incidence is much lower than the Western cancer incidence. In total it's significantly lower, and Japanese people live significantly longer because of the reduction in cancer risk. It's amazing how Japan is very different in cancer statistics than everywhere else. While perhaps some of it is racial, on the whole it's not, because when the Japanese move to new environments, they adapt very quickly to the cancer risk of the new environment, usually by the second generation, which makes one suspect that it's all, or mainly, in the diet. It probably reflects a combination of lifestyle and diet. It's not genetics.

– Professor Karol Sikora, Professor of Cancer Medicine
Imperial College School of Medicine
former Chief, World Health Organization Cancer Programme

DAY 6

HOW THE JAPANESE DIET COMPARES WITH THE UK DIET

How is the Japanese diet different from the UK diet?

Take a look at these figures from the United Nations, which give a rough estimate of the daily per-person calorie supply for both countries, and remember that 1980 was the year when the Japanese government considers the national diet achieved a state of 'nutritional balance':

The Japan Diet History
Supply of Calories Per Day Per Person

	Japan			UK		
	1961	1980	2003	1961	1980	2003
Vegetable products	2230	2203	2199	2015	1924	2393
Animal products	238	518	569	1275	1236	1057
Total	**2468**	**2721**	**2768**	**3290**	**3160**	**3450**

Animal key products:

Beef	5	15	27	74	66	64
Pork	9	59	84	266	275	244
Poultry	5	34	53	24	50	108
Fish	112	176	172	27	21	37
Milk	35	94	106	356	333	355
Eggs	35	65	76	58	54	46

	Japan				**UK**		
	1961	1980	2003		1961	1980	2003
Butter	3	11	14		178	120	67
Animal Fats	14	26	12		4	7	79
Vegetable key products:							
Rice	1150	780	610		12	22	56
Wheat	240	326	364		730	602	772
Soya Beans	106	93	97		0	0	0
Vegetables (various)	51	60	59		30	41	45
Sweet Potatoes, Yams	83	18	19		0	0	0
Beans, Peas, Pulses	36	21	18		28	28	40
Onions	7	10	11		5	8	11
Tomatoes	1	5	5		5	7	13
Potatoes	52	46	42		182	197	216
Fruits	34	55	52		74	70	114
Sugar and Sweeteners	173	322	271		513	427	401
Soya bean oil	31	108	137		20	113	112
Rapeseed oil	23	79	140		1	62	161
Corn oil	0	14	19		3	8	9

Do you notice the most striking differences?

• Japanese people eat 682 fewer calories per day than people in the UK.

• Japanese people eat more vegetable products as a proportion of their diet and may eat a greater variety of vegetables.

• Japanese people eat over four times more fish than people in the UK.

• Despite the increasing Westernisation of the Japanese diet, Japanese people eat less than half of the beef and almost one-third the amount of pork than people in the UK.

• Japanese people eat over 10 times more rice than people in the UK.

• Japanese people eat soya bean products as part of their diet in the form of soy sauce, tofu, edamame soya beans and natto (fermented soya beans), while people in the UK eat very little.

- Japanese people eat much less sugar than people in the UK.
- People in the UK consume much more butter, milk, potatoes and fruit.
- Japanese people have been using more of the healthy rapeseed cooking oil for a longer time than people in the UK, while people in the UK today are using six times more animal fat in their cooking.

The most intriguing point – Japanese people eat many of the same basic types of foods as people in the UK. But what's different is the quantity, the balance and the variety of food.

Dr Ann Yelmokas McDermott, Ph.D, is a research scientist at Tufts University, US Department of Agriculture Human Nutrition Research Center, in Boston. She told us:
Japanese and Asian cuisines are visually pleasing, flavorful, have lots of different spices and herbs and variety to pizzazz up the food so you don't have a monotonous diet.

Both the Asian and Mediterranean diets are plant-based and incorporate real food with healthy oils and moderate-sized portions that are high in fibre. Give me real foods and whole foods and healthy foods instead of packaged things. Go back to nature. Eat your colours.

Traditional Asian diets are plant-based. The animal protein source is usually the condiment to the meal as opposed to the American way, where half the plate is the steak and the other half is the fries. It's an accent to the meal but it's not the meal. The rice and veggies are the majority of the meal, with slivers of meat or a few shrimp or some fish. Often in America, the meal is the big piece of meat.

If you have a bowl of rice and veggies and some fish, the more complex the meal becomes in composition and chemical structure, and the longer you'll feel satisfied and full.

DAY 7

OPEN YOUR MIND TO THE JAPAN DIET ATTITUDE

The Japan Diet is, first and foremost, a new attitude.

It is an attitude that says the keys to a long, healthy life and long-term weight loss are balanced, sustained, nutritious eating and a physically active lifestyle.

It's time to revert back to the definition of 'diet' as our ancestors and grandparents knew it.

Let's start by truly understanding the word 'diet'.

In one leading dictionary, the second definition of the word is 'a course of food selected with reference to a particular state of health, prescribed allowance of food, regimen prescribed'.

That's how we now think of diets: a fixed allowance, a prescribed regimen. In other words, something you go on and then go off of, with limits, deprivation, rules, cravings and inevitably, failure. No wonder Dr Frankie Phillips, of the British Dietetic Association, said, 'The whole concept of a diet is not conducive to a healthy lifestyle.'

But it turns out that this bad idea has hijacked the number one definition of the word diet, which is very different: 'Course of living or nourishment, what is eaten and drunk habitually, food, victuals, fare.' Notice the difference – a 'course of living' rather than just a 'course of food.'

Now, these words I like! 'Eat'. 'Drink'. 'Food'. 'Fare'. 'Live and be nourished'. The best part is 'habitually'. To me it means something we do normally and naturally throughout our lives.

That's what a good diet, a healthy diet, should be: a lifetime of lean, healthy, delicious eating – with plenty of room for celebration, indulgence and joy.

Let's adopt a new diet attitude, you and I together, the Japan Diet Attitude:

Fad Diet Attitude	The Japan Diet Attitude
Prescribed regimen	A course of life
'I'm going on a diet.'	'I will eat to enjoy life and good health.'
Fast weight loss from extreme changes	Healthy weight loss from small, gradual changes
Forbidden foods, manipulation, elimination of food groups, or a single food or theory	Balance, moderation and variety, healthy eating from all food groups
Diet advice from testimonials, anecdotes, unsubstantiated theories	Evidence-based nutrition information
Fat is bad – carbs are bad	Healthy fats and healthy carbs are crucial to good health and heathy weight
Calorie obsession	Calorie awareness
Quantity	Quality
One-dimensional	Multi-dimensional
Forced	Enjoyed
Food is the enemy, a source of guilt, shame, failure and anger	Food is about life, celebration and joy

If you agree with the statements on the right-hand side, why don't you grab a pen and tick them off on the page. Then make a photocopy and stick it on your refrigerator or kitchen notice board.

Prof. Robert Vogel, MD, is a Cardiologist, Professor of Medicine and Director of Vascular Biology, at the University of Maryland School of Medicine. He told us:
The Japanese diet is easily as good or better than the highly touted Mediterranean diet. Whereas both Japanese and Mediterraneans have less heart disease, the Japanese live quite a bit longer.

Foremost are the portion sizes in the Japanese diet, which are clearly less than ours.

Their diet is substantially fruit/vegetable/complex carbohydrate based, whereas ours is animal/simple sugar based. Approximately three-fourths of the current American dietary calories come from fat and sugar.

The Japanese have learned to eat a low-calorie density diet which prevents hunger. Their love for fish probably plays an important role, as does the great expense of their beef. Even considering fruits and vegetables, fish is probably the best documented healthy food.

An interesting lesson from the Japanese is that they eat a relatively large amount of rice, but are not fat (in the past) and have a great lifespan. So much for the Atkins' concept.

Like all good culinary societies, the Japanese traditionally dine rather than scoff down their food, although that is changing. Their food is wonderfully 'presented' rather than wrapped in a cardboard box.

We know from the NiHonSan (Nippon-Japan, Honolulu, San Fransisco) study that Japanese genes play little if any role in their longevity since Japanese moving to Honolulu or San Francisco develop the same heart disease rates and longevity as do locals.

The Japan Diet 'Red Flag' – too much sodium

A big problem with both the Japanese and UK national diets is they contain too much sodium. The FSA recommends that adults should eat no more than 6 g of salt – or about 2.5 g (2,500 milligrams) of sodium – per day (about 1 teaspoonful) to reduce the risk of high blood pressure and related heart disease, kidney disease and stroke.

In Japan, adults eat about 12 g of salt per day. Some of the leading sources are soy sauce, pickled vegetables and salted dried fish.

In the UK, adults are eating an average of 9.5 g of salt per day, or 60 per cent more than they should. Surprisingly, much of the salt in the UK diet comes from processed foods, takeaway foods and restaurant meals. Huge amounts of salt are hidden in fast food, breakfast cereals, soups, sauces, bagels, bread, biscuits, salad dressings and ready meals, to name just a few items. Only 10 to 15 per cent comes from the salt added to the cooking or at the dinner table.

Remember, salt and sodium aren't exactly the same thing: a little less than half the volume of salt is sodium. You multiply the sodium figure by 2.5 to work out the amount of salt. 6 g of salt equals about 2.5 g, or 2,500 milligrams of sodium. Most food labels list the sodium content. According to the FSA:

This is A LOT of salt or sodium:
- 1.25 g salt or more per 100 g, or
- 0.5 g sodium or more per 100 g

This is A LITTLE salt or sodium – try to choose these:
- 0.25 g salt or less per 100 g, or
- 0.1 g sodium or less per 100 g

Ten Tips for Reducing Sodium
These are adapted from the FSA, Heart UK and the US National Institutes of Health:
1. Make the change slowly – switch to low-sodium eating over a few weeks or months to give your taste buds time to adjust.
2. On food labels, look for the sodium content in milligrams (mg), or grams (g), and keep a note of how it adds up through your day. Try to keep your daily sodium intake below 2.5 g, or 2,500 milligrams of sodium.
3. Try to get out of the habit of automatically shaking salt onto your food at the table.

4. Choose low- or reduced-sodium, or no-salt-added versions of foods, condiments and tinned vegetables.

5. In cooking and at the table, instead of salt, flavour food with black pepper, spices, herbs, lemon, lime, salt-free seasoning blends, garlic, or these Japanese- and Asian-style favourites: white or black sesame seeds, ginger, seaweed or seven-spice powder.

6. Choose ready-to-eat breakfast cereals that are lower in sodium.

7. Cook rice, pasta and hot cereals without salt. Cut back on instant or flavoured rice, pasta and cereal mixes, which usually have added salt.

8. Choose 'convenience' foods and ready meals that are lower in sodium.

9. When eating out, ask how much sodium is used in food preparation. Most restaurants will accommodate low-sodium requirements.

10. Cut down on foods that are high in salt, like anchovies, bacon, cheese, chips (if salt is added), crisps, olives, pickles, pretzels, salted and dry roasted nuts, sausages, smoked meat and fish and tinned and packet soups.

I suggest that you always choose lower-sodium options for highly salted foods such as miso (which is made from fermented soya beans), soy sauce and teriyaki sauce, and even then, you should use them in small amounts. I think soy sauce should be used sparingly on food and in cooking, even the lower-sodium varieties. On a piece of sushi, for example, just a drop or two of lower-sodium soy sauce is all you need.

DAY 8

REACH FOR REALISTIC, ATTAINABLE GOALS

You don't have to go through this journey of 'The Japan Diet' alone. I encourage you to reach out to partners and allies. Do it with your spouse, partner, family members, or your close friends. This is a golden opportunity for everyone to get involved, to prepare and eat delicious, healthy food together.

If you're really serious about getting to a healthy weight, I hope the first thing you'll do is visit your GP or a registered dietitian to work out a healthy eating plan that's customised for you and your family, with precise, in-depth advice, taking into account any personal medical conditions, medication and nutritional supplements.

Discuss with your doctor, your dietitian, your partner and your family everything you are learning about healthy eating in general and how you can put this knowledge into action.

By exploring The Japan Diet with your family and friends, you can share shopping tips, shortcuts and recipes, support each other and ask each other questions. You'll enjoy dining out together and you'll enjoy the shared experiences.

The Japan Diet might *not* be for you if:
- You're not open to an entirely new attitude towards food.
- You think you can absolutely never live without constant, regular doses of fizzy drinks, deep-fried foods, greasy food, cakes, heavy creamy sauces, piles of biscuits, cookies and doughnuts and fast food.

- You're addicted to yo-yo dieting.
- You're looking for a miracle crash diet or instant weight loss.

If you have an unhealthy diet, I would like to see you move towards these goals:
- Change the way you feel about food.
- Change the way you buy food.
- Change the way you look at food.
- Change the way you prepare food.
- Change the way you eat.
- Fall in love with food in a new way.
- Feel absolutely fantastic and totally positive.
- Be healthy over the long term.

The Japan Diet involves a gradual move towards the goal of lifelong, permanent healthy eating and lifestyle habits. Please stop and ask yourself if you really want to achieve this goal. Are you ready to make some physical, emotional and intellectual shifts? Will you allocate enough time, effort and energy to change your habits?

What is your most important weight-loss goal?
Examples:
- 'I want to feel healthy and fantastic.'
- 'I want to fit into my sexy black dress and tight jeans.'
- 'I want to chase my kids around the block, hike up a hill with my partner or walk up a flight of stairs without getting winded.'

Write your goal down here. If you have two or three goals, write them down too.

1 _____

2 _____

3 _____

Write down the top three reasons why you think you might *not* achieve this goal:

1 _____

2 _____

3 _____

Write down exactly how you will overcome each of the reasons listed above:

1 _____

2 _____

3 _____

Write down the top three *excuses* you may give for not achieving this goal:

1 _____

2 _____

3 _____

Write down how you will overcome each excuse listed above:

1 _____

2 _____

3 _____

Are you 100 per cent committed?
Tick below:

No? _____ Then read on, and come back and answer these questions again when you think you are ready.

Yes? _____ Then let's go!

While everyone is different, many experts agree that a key to healthy long-term weight loss is to pursue a series of small steps and gradual changes. 'Pick one or two changes to start with,' suggests

Cindy Moore, director of nutrition therapy at the Cleveland Clinic Foundation. 'Once the changes have become habits, which usually happens in about two to four weeks, then try adding one or two more. In six to 12 months, you'll find that you've made substantial changes.'

Remember – a weight-loss target of 0.5–1 kg (1–2 lb) a week is considered to be a realistic, achievable goal. That's the rate at which I lost all my excess weight in Tokyo, and I can tell you it felt natural and sustainable.

But you can see good concrete results on a slower timetable, too. 'The key is moderation,' wrote Dr John J. Whyte and Dr Robert N. Marting in the May 2005 issue of *Patient Care*. 'Small, stepwise changes can have a big impact. For instance, reducing intake by as little as 100 calories per day translates into 10 lb [4.5 kg] of weight loss in a year.'

As a next step, let's see how you measure up today. Gather up:
- a pencil or pen
- a notepad
- a tape measure
- an accurate scale
- a full size mirror and
- a camera or video camera – so you can see yourself in 360 degrees and keep a visual record of your progress over time.

Self assessment: how I'm doing right now

Today's date _____
Age _____
Weight _____
I feel: 1 2 3 4 5 6 7 8 9 10 (circle one number: 1 is terrible; 10 is fantastic)
Body Mass Index (BMI) _____
To calculate your BMI online, go to www.eatwell.gov.uk and search for BMI Calculator. It's easy, all you need to know is your height and weight. If you can't get online, take your weight (in kilograms) and divide this by your height (in metres, squared).

Here's how the British Dietetic Association defines (BDA) different BMI ranges:

- A BMI of less than 18.5 kg/m^2 indicates you are underweight. You may need to gain weight.
- A BMI of 19 to 24.9 kg/m^2 is regarded as a healthy weight. You should aim to stay that weight.
- A BMI of 25 to 29 kg/m^2 is defined as overweight. It's a good idea to lose some weight for your health's sake, or at least aim to prevent further weight gain.
- A BMI of over 30 kg/m^2 is defined as fat and means your health is at risk. Losing weight will improve your health. (This BMI is also the WHO's international definition of 'obese'.)
- A BMI of over 35 kg/m^2 means you should visit your GP for a health check-up, as you may need specialist help to manage your weight and health. This is especially important before taking up any new exercise.

It's important to bear in mind, though, that the BDA says that the BMI is not always a good reflection of body fatness. A very muscular person might have a high BMI even though 'their body fat is at a healthy level, as muscle weighs more than fat'.

Additionally, the FSA points out that the BMI is only a guide aimed at healthy adults and is 'not suitable for children, young people or older people'. A better guide is your waist measurement, as people who store excess fat around their middle are at greater risk of health problems such as heart disease, high blood pressure and Type 2 diabetes.

Write down your waist measurement _____

To measure your waist, find the bottom of your ribs and the top of your hips, and measure around your middle at a point mid-way between these two (for many people this will be the tummy button). This BDA chart shows those who are at increased and high risk of heart disease, high blood pressure and diabetes:

Waist measurement for adult:	Increased risk	High risk
European men	94 cm (37 in)	102 cm (40 in)
Asian men	90 cm (36 in)	—
European and Asian women	80 cm (32 in)	88 cm (35 in)

Where I want to go

Now that you know where you are, it's time to set realistic goals for yourself. You won't achieve everything you want all at once, so use the chart opposite to set your goals as a series of milestones. In the 'I want to feel . . .' column write down a number; 1 is terrible; 10 is fantastic.

When you pass each milestone, do the self-assessment, as before, and also report to your GP or dietitian as necessary, so that you can monitor how you're doing. Be honest with yourself. At the same time, forgive yourself for any setbacks and plateaux – they're perfectly human and completely normal.

Japan Diet Tip: Keep a Food Journal

In addition to absorbing the new insights, writing down your thoughts in the book, taking the small steps day by day and measuring your progress long-term, I recommend that you keep a food journal.

Clare MacAvilly, of the Medical Research Council, suggests that you 'write down what you eat over the course of the day, really monitor what you're eating'. For some people, keeping a food journal works quite well, she reports, since 'they're quite horrified when they realize that over the course of the day they've been snacking so much!' The journal will help you see if you are following the principles of the Japan Diet, and also might help you identify the eating habits you didn't even know you had!

On page 44, there's a sample food diary sheet from the US National Institutes of Health. Why don't you make copies of this and fill it out each day for the next week or two. It should help you zero in on how you feel and how you act when it comes to food, and may identify some easy steps for improvement.

The Japan Diet Healthy Progress Chart

	Date	Weight	BMI	Waist measurement	I want to feel . . .
Goal: Two Weeks from Now					
Actual: Two Weeks					
Goal: One Month					
Actual: One Month					
Goal: Two Months					
Actual: Two Months					
Goal: Three Months					
Actual: Three Months					
Goal: Six Months					
Actual: Six Months					
Goal: Nine Months					
Actual: Nine Months					
Goal: One Year from Today					
Actual: One Year					

FOOD DIARY

Date

Time	Food	Feelings

DAY 9

STEP INTO A BEAUTIFUL WORLD – RIGHT AROUND THE CORNER

I recently came across the story of a strapping Italian man named Alessandro Valignano. He set off for Japan a couple of hundred years ago to launch a new branch of the Catholic Church. It seems he was amazed by what he found there, and pretty baffled.

The people walked around in kimonos and flip-flops. The language seemed not only incomprehensible, but absolutely unlearnable. The standard meal was a bowl of rice, a piece of fish and some veggies, served on tableware that looked imported from another planet.

Writing about his trip, the Jesuit cleric marvelled, 'They have rites and customs so different from those of all other nations that it seems they deliberately try to be unlike any other people. The things they do in this respect are beyond imagining and it may truly be said that Japan is a world the reverse of Europe.'

Does the idea of Japanese food and customs sometimes seem a bit intimidating to you, too? I don't blame you. At first, it must seem like a mystery. There are some strange-sounding dishes and some ideas that are kind of upside-down from what you grew up with. But the basic logic of the Japanese diet is easy to understand and easy to see.

The lessons of The Japan Diet are all around you and possibly just around the corner, at your local Japanese formal restaurant, noodle shop or sushi takeaway. The UK has already fallen deeply in love with Japanese food, and hundreds of Japanese-themed restaurants have popped up so there is now one in practically every city and major town. They range from bustling conveyor-belt sushi emporiums, eateries serving casual noodle bowls or haute cuisine fusion to ultra-authentic places. English chefs in all kinds of restaurants are experimenting with Japanese ingredients, such as wasabi, miso, ponzu dipping sauce, and yuzu – the sharply tangy citrus flavouring.

You can now get world-class Japanese food in Edinburgh, Manchester, Leeds, Birmingham, Cardiff and all around the UK. In London, the city anointed by one journal as 'the most exciting restaurant city in the world', you'll find an embarrassment of Japanese food riches. In 2005, *Tatler* proclaimed super-chic Zuma as the best restaurant in London. In 2006, the Wagamama noodle chain was named the most popular restaurant in the *Zagat London Restaurants Guide*. 'Japanese cuisine could soon be as common on our high streets as fish and chips,' predicted Simon Beckett in *The Independent*.

I read that Tesco is selling more sushi these days than British cheese sandwiches, and you can also pick up a sushi pack at Boot's, Sainsbury's, Waitrose and Marks & Spencer. Words like ramen (noodles in soup), sashimi (fresh sliced fish) and gyoza (dumplings, see page 194 for a recipe) now co-exist in the national food consciousness along with bangers and mash and bubble and squeak.

At lunchtime, sushi shops like Itsu and Yo! Sushi are bustling with office workers. 'We're talking big,' declared writer Alex Renton in the 26 February 2006 *Observer Food Monthly*. 'Sushi is the Japanese tapas, sushi is the new pizza, sushi is the sandwich of the 21st century.' The reason, he explained: 'It's healthy, Zen, stylish.'

My office is in the middle of New York's fashion district and at lunchtime you'll often find me at a terrific little sushi takeaway shop, Norimaki, nearby. They make your sushi rolls fresh – right in front of you. The food is fast, filling and doesn't knock me into a sleepy stupor like a heavy cheese- or mayo-drenched lunch will.

There's a nutritional reason for this 'sushi effect', according to dietitian Jacqui Lowden, of the University Hospital of Wales, in Cardiff. She said, 'It's low calorie but it's carbohydrate, so it's filling, which means you're less likely to snack in that mid-afternoon dip.' A sushi lunch is relatively low in fat and, she added, 'you have the protein as it tends to be fish and also a little bit of veg'. Ms Lowden called sushi 'a healthier option' compared with packets of sandwiches loaded with mayonnaise and other toppings.

To see The Japan Diet in action, let's take a field trip.

Why don't we splurge a bit on ourselves?

Let's pay a visit to a great Japanese restaurant like, let's say, Matsuri in London's High Holborn. Here, the décor is exquisite, the food is super-fresh and the atmosphere is chic. It has a spacious main dining room, an elegant sushi counter and a special room downstairs reserved for 'teppan-yaki', which, very loosely translated, means fresh ingredients grilled before your eyes by a knife-wielding master showman-chef.

If you look around the restaurant, you can see the main pillars of Japanese food all under one roof: fish, vegetables, rice, soya, tea and fruit. What looks good? How about appetisers like edamame soya beans, chawan-mushi (savoury steamed egg custard with assorted ingredients) marinated salmon, or agedashi-tofu (golden deep-fried tofu in a sweet soy sauce).

For the next course, perhaps assorted sashimi along with miso soup and wholegrain brown genmai rice, and a main course of grilled sea bream or prawn sauté, followed by some soul-quenching green tea. There are more Westernised dishes here, too, and many Japanese restaurants in the West tailor their menu to satisfy local preferences, for example, by adding more meat-based dishes and having larger portions than those of their counterparts in Japan.

What many of the dishes here have in common with each other, and with good Japanese food all over the world, is a relatively healthy balance of foods, cooking styles and portions, all of which can demonstrate some important lessons, even before you learn to cook a single Japanese-style dish.

Japan Diet field trip

This week, take a research excursion into a Japanese-style restaurant in your town, to familiarise yourself with some of the basic themes of Japanese-style eating. The best place to visit would be a restaurant that serves authentic, traditional Japanese dishes, but you can also see the lessons of The Japan Diet in action at a good Japanese noodle shop or sushi restaurant:

• Take a few minutes to consider the menu, the portion sizes and the balance of foods offered. Think of what good, easy steps you could apply to your daily food life.

• Take time to notice *what isn't there* – like massive desserts and huge doses of saturated fat.

• Study how the food is arranged on a plate and notice the tableware and composition. How large or small is the plate? How large or small is each piece of food presented? Are there any natural garnishes, such as a maple leaf added to the plate to heighten the sense of season? Next time you're entertaining your friends, you could add your own garnishes to your plates to add a beautiful accent of nature like this.

Prof. Mike Lean is Chairman of the Department of Human Nutrition at the University of Glasgow and Consultant Physician at Glasgow Royal Infirmary. He is a leading authority on obesity, health and nutrition. He explained:

What does sushi mean to a nutritionist? Well, the vast variety of sushi and other Japanese foods is itself interesting.

One of the nutritional hazards of the fast food revolution arises from its sameness. Variety is a good measure of nutritional excellence. It ensures the nutrients we know we need, and many we do not know about, are more likely to be supplied by a range of foods like sushi than by the same old burger day after day.

A sushi meal is surprisingly filling, but provides only about 300–400 kcals. Its slightly glutinous consistency makes the rice chewy, and interspacing eight pieces of sushi with ginger turns it into eight small, different meals. Eating with chopsticks also makes 300 kcals go a bit further than usual, so if your weight is a problem – and remember, obesity is rare in Japan – sushi is for you.

Japanese cookery is big on freshness, using produce in season and sourced locally, where possible. The balance of nutrients in Japanese food is obviously not too bad, since the Japanese are the most long-lived race on earth. The emphasis is on vegetables and some fruit. Particularly beneficial are the omega-3 fatty acids and iodine in fish, with very little saturated fats – before the advent of fast food, meat in Japan was a rare and expensive delicacy.

Japanese food is fun and eating it is fun, without the need for cheap gimmicks like plastic toys. Kids love it too.

SEE THE BEAUTY OF MINDFUL EATING

Not long ago, I experienced one of the most deeply 'mindful' eating experiences of my life. My parents, husband and I had spent the day hiking up Mount Takao, one of the small mountains that are closest to Tokyo, about an hour north of the city by train. We found ourselves in the little detached dining room of a wonderful restaurant called Ukai-Toriyama, which serves Japanese country-style meals. Their speciality is charcoal-grilled free-range organic chicken, which they raise on a farm.

● ● ● ● ●

The beauty of Ukai-Toriyama is its setting, in a wooded valley graced with flowers and rushing streams. A kimono-clad woman escorts us to a thatch-roofed wooden hut adorned inside with tatami mats, an exquisite vase and three stems of a seasonal flower. There is an oversized window overlooking a river, a water-mill, carefully trimmed bushes and ranges of mountains in the distance.

The lady in the kimono welcomes us, takes our drinks order and walks away. A man knocks on the door and enters with a small bucket of charcoals. He places a few black-red charcoals on the brazier with a pair of long metal chopsticks, sets up a grill tray over them and walks away. The hostess returns with our drinks. She then starts bringing our meal course by course.

It is a slow-motion procession of many small dishes that are arranged and served like miniature works of art, in a theatrical banquet that unfolds in a leisurely fashion over the course of a few hours.

The appetiser is a handful of mountain potatoes sliced like angel hair pasta served with broth made from sea vegetables and fish. Then comes a slice of tender duck with a chunk of simmered summer gourd, followed by clear soup with tiny chicken meat balls.

Every time a course is brought in, the waitress explains what we are about to enjoy, and sometimes how we are supposed to eat it. We stop talking and listen to her while intently looking at the course in front of us. Sometimes we ask her a question or two. Where was the Ayu river-fish caught? A nearby river? After a bite or mouthful, we exchange remarks on the food, and often on its presentation.

I see my mother making a mental note as to how she would arrange a similar dish next time at home. The whole experience is pristine, elegant and even relaxing, and not stifling or formal at all. Time slows down and eventually stops at a place like this. The outer world beyond the valley recedes into nothingness. Our vision is soaked in the tranquil scenery and we feel like we're floating in the valley, rather than sitting in a room. We are cocooned in this tiny hut, just us and the meal.

Every 15 minutes or so, the waitress shuffles up to the door of the hut, brings us the next course and refreshes our tea. Every time she reaches the hut, she puts down the tray, takes off her sandals, slides the door open, walks into the house and kneels by the table to arrange the dishes. She moves so quietly, we hardly notice her except to note how very pleasant she is. She helps us charcoal-grill the chicken. Sizzling sounds over the hot orange coals suggest the climax of the meal is nearing.

Chicken chunks on skewers are dipped into the restaurant's original barbecue sauce, and a sweet aroma wafts over the grill, encouraging our appetites. The outer layer of the chicken turns crusty and light brown. My dad turns the skewers and examines the 'doneness' of the chicken. When they are crisp and golden on the outside, he says to Billy, 'Bill-san, this is ready,' and gestures my husband to bring over his plate. I reach out for a skewer, too. A piece of chicken is smoky-crunchy outside, juicy inside and altogether hearty.

A bowl of barley and rice arrives, topped with grated mountain potatoes and accompanied by a bowl of miso soup and a few slivers of pickled vegetables on a tiny plate. This is the final act of the main course. Fruit and tea complete the banquet.

After the meal, the charcoal man returns, takes the grill tray aside and ceremonially smoothes out the ashes in the brazier with a fan-shaped spatula that has a wave pattern at the bottom, creating even-width lines in the ashes.

• • • • •

What was so special about this meal was not just the very attractive and delicious food and the stunning view of nature through the window, but the feeling of a family moment that was shared and savoured to its fullest.

This is traditional Japanese dining at its core, at its purest and most dazzling, a style that takes the concept of 'slow food' and pushes it to an intoxicating limit.

The experience is a showcase of one of the classic bits of Japanese food wisdom, which says that having a meal is an aesthetic, almost theatrical experience. You don't eat just to fill your belly in a hurry but to please your visual, aromatic, textural senses, as well as your taste buds.

There is nothing exclusively Japanese about 'mindful eating' and on any given day in Japan you'll find millions of people quickly slurping bowlfuls of noodles without even lifting their heads, or wolfing down cheeseburgers without devoting much thought to the beauty of nature or family traditions.

But something we all share in the traditions of our families and ancestors is the notion that food should be enjoyed slowly and fully with the people we love. It is an endangered tradition, as we skip meals and eat on the run or in front of the TV.

I think it's time we reconnected with mindful eating. Mindful eating not only feels great, there are experts who are convinced it can help us lose weight. Like many theories in the diet and nutrition field, there isn't yet much in the way of rock-solid research to be found on the subject of mindful eating, and some studies have not found weight-control benefits for such 'mindful' practices of slow eating, meal-pausing or extra chewing.

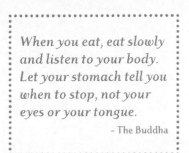

When you eat, eat slowly and listen to your body. Let your stomach tell you when to stop, not your eyes or your tongue.

– The Buddha

But one fairly large recent Japanese study of 4,400 people found a direct link between the speed of eating and a person's body mass index. Slow eaters had a low rise in weight over time and the fastest eaters had the biggest weight gain. The researchers' conclusion, reported at the 2005 meeting of the North American Association for the Study of Obesity, was that 'eating fast may lead to obesity, independent of energy intake or other lifestyle factors in middle-aged, non-diabetic men and women'.

Dr Peter Fox, MD, of the University of Texas, has conducted laboratory experiments with groups of adults, testing the effects of different eating speeds. He concluded that 'eating slowly may provide more time for the feeling of fullness to occur – especially in the obese, where fullness signals are slower'.

It takes at least 10 or 15 minutes for your stomach's 'fullness' signals to reach your brain, according to Dr James O. Hill, MD, director of the Center for Nutrition at the University of Colorado. 'Eat too quickly,' he said, 'and you're almost guaranteed to overeat.' Dr Ann Yelmokas McDermott, of the USDA Human Nutrition Research Center, at Tufts University, in Boston, agreed, explaining, 'You have to give your body time to understand.'

And Dr Toshiie Sakata, MD, a Japanese obesity expert, said he believes that some 80 per cent of obese people are rapid eaters who eat big mouthfuls of food. He sees the vegetables, rice and fibre in the traditional Japanese diet as helping people chew more, which he said is 'well-known to suppress food intake' and speed up the breakdown of fat. The Japanese diet, he argues, 'is quite effective not only for weight reduction but for long-term maintenance of reduced weight loss'.

> The Japanese tend to be less 'unconscious' in their eating – that is, they are less likely to eat in front of the TV or at the movies. They also tend to be more aware of their food environment, and place more value on the aesthetics of their food: ambience, preparation, freshness and taste. There is a clear lesson for Westerners: stop eating on the run, stop eating unconsciously and stop eating indiscriminately, as in highly processed, super-size portions of fast food and junk food.
>
> – Professor Steven R. Hawks
> Professor of Health Science, Brigham Young University

Mindful eating begins where you buy your food. The city I live in, New York, can be a wall-to-wall unhealthy food trap, and I bet your town is too. If I am not mindful about what I eat, I could easily load up on the wrong foods and quickly go back to being overweight, if not obese, and feeling unhealthy and unwell.

I could step out of our apartment in the morning, stop at one of the pavement coffee stalls and grab a glazed doughnut and a cup of coffee with milk and sugar. Or I could scoff a sugary corn muffin at the office while I check my e-mails.

It would be really easy for me to take a cab to the office every day instead of walking 20 blocks each way, and for lunch get an oversized sandwich from the deli filled with mayonnaise, salt and extra layers of roast beef.

For dinner, I could grab a saturated fat-soaked 'curbside takeaway' from a neighbourhood steakhouse and gobble down the entire meal in a few minutes out of a paper bag in front of TV. On top of all that, I could stock our larder and fridge with a bag of brownies and a bucket of chocolate chip ice cream for midnight snacks.

This kind of impulse to eat and drink mindlessly is really easy to develop, don't you think? It's blind eating, the opposite of mindful eating.

I believe it's perfectly OK and healthy to yield to your craving for super-indulgent foods, as long as you are mindful about it and make it occasional rather than a daily habit.

Mindful shopping and eating is a way of navigating through the dangers of our 'obesinogenic' world. No matter how simple your meal might be, you can practise mindful eating, find its beauty and eventually feel it deep inside of you.

Be mindful – open your eyes before you open your mouth. Be smart – be conscious of what you select to eat and demand delicious, healthy food for your body and soul.

Stop blind eating and engage yourself in the beauty of mindful eating. It can become second nature for you.

Naomi's Top Tips for Mindful Eating

When shopping and dining:

1. Open your eyes before you walk into a store or restaurant. Ask yourself if this is the sort of place that would serve the kinds of food you want to eat. Once inside, visualise the lessons of healthy eating and The Japan Diet and order your meal accordingly.
2. When you shop for groceries or a ready meal, be mindful of what you're buying.
3. Don't look away when your hand automatically grabs a big bag of cookies, crisps or a tub of ice cream. Stop and think. Connect your brain to your hand actions and be mindful of your choices.
4. Take a second to consider if the choice you're making is going to make you feel good in a healthy way or an unhealthy way, right after the meal and for the long term.
5. When your body feels like a magnet for junk food:
   - Forgive yourself – don't feel guilty about the urge.
   - Stop and think if you really must have it.

- Stop and try to remember the last time you had a not-so-healthy meal.
- Think of long-term inconveniences to your health and how you feel.

At the dinner table:

1. Slow down the pace of the meal, take your time and enjoy yourself. Don't be a speed eater.
2. Don't eat meals while watching TV or otherwise distracted – focus on your food.
3. Drink in your food with all your senses – sight, smell, feel, taste and even sound.
4. Eat with your eyes. Take a moment to consider how pleasing and beautiful your food is and how lucky you are to have it.
5. Appreciate your food's colours, textures and aromas and the complex sensations it creates in your mouth.
6. Savour each mouthful in small, luxurious bites and chew your food well.
7. Let the beauty of food slowly take over the rest of you.
8. Give your brain enough time to know when you've had enough.
9. Eat until you're satisfied – not until you're stuffed.

DAY 11

LIBERATE YOUR DISHES AND HUMANISE YOUR PORTIONS

In the UK, many people are falling into an 'energy imbalance'. They're eating too many calories per day and not moving around enough to burn them off. It is a fundamental, relentless process that ends up with you carrying around extra weight on your body.

The country I live in, the USA, has sadly become the world capital of energy imbalance, with more and more people eating hundreds of calories more per day than they work off.

One reason is that portion sizes have exploded. Twenty years ago, a typical American blueberry muffin serving size was 210 calories. Today it's 500. The typical cola has risen from 85 calories to 250. French fries, or chips, have gone from 210 calories to over 600.

Consider what happened recently to some Japanese visitors to the USA.

One day at the Carnegie Deli in Las Vegas, a 157 kg (24 st 9 lb) sumo wrestler named Futeno came face-to-face with a pastrami on rye sandwich. He could not believe what he saw.

It was so huge, so vast and so belly-bustlingly massive that the visiting athlete could not wrap his fingers around it. 'Is that the size for the American people, too?' he marvelled. 'Of course, it's too big.'

Not far away, one of his colleagues gazed upon the all-you-can-eat buffet at the Mandalay Bar Resort and Casino and said, 'Everything is so big here, it makes me feel small.'

Think about it – portion sizes that are too big for sumo wrestlers!

Have you ever had a 'stomach freeze?' You know how it feels when you've scoffed down a big greasy fast-food meal and a few minutes later not only are you full, but you're so stuffed you want to untie your belt and roll around on the floor, gasping for air? I think that feeling has started to become normal and we misconstrue this crazy over-fullness as the sign of having had a satisfying meal.

As competition among food and restaurant companies has driven them to offer 'value meals' and 'super-size' portions, we've lost control of portion sizes. We've got used to sandwiches and pancakes and burgers so big that they're really more suitable for giant beasts in the fields, rather than people. I say, let's liberate our dishes by giving them room to breathe and not burying them in food. Let's bring back human-size portions.

There appears to be a direct connection between the amount of food that's placed in front of us and the amount we over-eat. 'Studies show that people tend to passively overeat by about 25 per cent,' explained Professor James Hill, of the University of Colorado. 'In other words, three-quarters of the way through a big bowl of pasta, you may be perfectly satisfied. But if there's more in the bowl, you'll eat it.'

In Japan, however, the food portion sizes and the average daily supply of calories per person have managed to stay much lower and fairly constant, over the past few decades. The portions are smaller and the dishes themselves are, too. As Professor Marion Nestle, chairwoman of the department of nutrition at New York University wrote, 'The courses Japanese eat are like the little things you pass around on a cocktail platter before dinner.'

Japanese people are the world's Master Portion Controllers and luckily the idea of super-sizing in Japan has never caught on. Since much of Japan is mountain country, not suitable for crops or cattle, it's never had a huge over-abundance of food, and the Japanese food culture has become adept at celebrating and savouring relatively smaller volumes of food. The emphasis is on quality rather than quantity.

'Food is about more than just nutrients, it is about a whole way of life,' said Susan A. Jebb, PhD, RD, Head of Nutrition and Health

Research at the Medical Research Council in Cambridge. 'It seems to be that "valuing food" is an important part of the Japanese culture that helps to foster a degree of respect which encourages moderation.'

Traditionally, a Japanese food portion is served in a moderate size on its own individual small, pretty plate. In fact, there's really no main course as such, but a satisfying variety of tastes and textures in manageable sizes: rice in a rice bowl, miso soup in a soup bowl, simmered vegetables in a bowl or plate, sea vegetable salad with rice vinegar dressing in a little bowl, a fillet of fish on a plate. Dishes such as noodles with toppings in a delicious broth are served in bowls that are 10–20 per cent smaller than their Western counterparts.

I often go back for seconds and even thirds for some of my favourite dishes. But to me, having two or three servings of a modest portion is not as over-stuffing somehow as one serving of a huge pile of food, probably because the pace of the meal is slowed down. By spacing out between each serving, my brain knows when my stomach is full and when to stop eating, as we discussed in Mindful Eating on Day 10.

If you were to visit a Japanese home for dinner tonight, you'd feel right at home, and what you saw on the table would look much the same as your own. There would be a few small but important differences: there would be a pair of chopsticks and the dishes, plates and bowls would be much smaller than you're used to.

It's easy to apply the lessons of Japan-style portion control in your life right away, just by 'tweaking' the way you think about how your food should be laid out.

Japanised Western meal:
- Piece of lean meat, no gravy, on a small plate
- Side salad
- Piece of multigrain bread, no butter
- Big order of mixed vegetables on a medium plate
- Dessert: small piece of cake

Japan-style meal:
(Typical formula: a soup and three side dishes, plus a bowl of rice)
- Bowl of brown rice in its own small bowl
- Small bowl of miso soup or clear soup
- 85 g (3 oz) piece of fish on its own plate
- Spinach leaves with sesame dressing on its own dish
- Simmered mixed vegetables on its own dish
- Dessert: dish of mixed fruit and tiny bowl of green tea

How to Japan-style your portions

Japanese-style portion control is 'the iPod of food'. It concentrates the magnificent energy of food into a satisfying, pleasurable, convenient and compact size. Here are ten ideas to liberate your dishes, humanise your portions 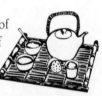 and restore the volume of the food you eat to the proper balance.

- Learn the correct portion sizes and proportions. The proper serving size of pasta or rice is only about the size of a tennis ball. The portion sizes you've got accustomed to could actually be three or four servings, with more calories, sugar and saturated fat than you realise. One 85 g (3 oz) portion of poultry or meat, for example, is about the size of a deck of cards, while restaurant steaks can range into several hundreds of grams.
- Give your food portions a trim. If you're eating 25 per cent too many excess calories a day, for example, cut down your portion sizes by a quarter.
- Boost your vegetables and salads. As a general rule, never be afraid to serve large portions of veggies that are prepared in a healthy way.
- Cook up a smaller, leaner portion of red meat and/or adding vegetables and pieces of tofu, for example, to your minced beef.
- For desserts and sweets, switch to serving smaller pieces on their own individual, smaller-size plates.

- Lighten your tableware. Bring your smaller plates and bowls to centre stage: bread, appetiser and condiments plates, small salad bowls and soup cups. Use them at every meal for individual servings of fish, veggies, tofu, rice and soup, and help yourself to multiple servings of veggies.

- When you buy new tableware, select smaller sizes. You can look into Asian-inspired tableware collections now being offered by a number of manufacturers and retailers, which feature East-meets-West designs and modest-size plates, dishes and bowls.

- Try some Japanese tableware for your home – it's like an Armani dress for your food. If you serve your usual food on Japanese tableware, you'll cut your portion sizes by at least a quarter, if not in half, and I think your food will look more beautiful. Japanese speciality shops offer fascinating selections of tableware from Japan, including stoneware, lacquerware and ceramic pieces.

- Remember that empty space is an important part of food presentation. Your plates don't have to be buried in food. Empty space brings elegance, harmony and balance to the plate.

- Add chopsticks to your table. Consider buying some wooden, bamboo or lacquered chopsticks as an optional utensil for your table (don't get plastic ones; they're too slippery to grab anything). They can require practice to get used to, but once you do, they're great for Japan-style eating. Chopsticks can help you to eat more slowly and take smaller bites, including when eating many of your own non-Japanese dishes.

Radically simple Japan Diet portion shortcut: the Bento Box

How would you like to:
- Do less washing up
- Make your food more deliciously beautiful
- And instantly and easily 'humanise' your portion sizes?

All you have to do is buy a Japan-style Bento Box for your meals at home.

A Bento Box is a portable container that carries a single meal, with anywhere from two to six little compartments for different foods. Bento Boxes are ubiquitous in Japan. You'll see them at schools, offices, restaurants, takeaway places, theatres, railway station kiosks, on long-distance trains and at picnic sites and sports arenas.

Their origin traces back 400 years to when people brought picnic-style meal boxes to outdoor parties and picnics. Today, Bento Boxes come in various materials and shapes; some are made of plastic and come with lids that make them leak free, even when they're tilted.

For a once-or-twice a week, super-easy alternative to using your usual tableware at home, you can buy a pretty medium-size plastic Bento Box for around £15, with a simulated red-and-black lacquerware finish. This is a durable modern plastic version of the traditional lacquerware Bento Box. It is dishwasher proof and has multiple food serving compartments.

I think the Bento Box is a brilliant invention. I love serving food in my plastic Bento Boxes at home. They allow you to pack several different foods in one beautiful serving tray without the flavours getting mixed up together and you only have to carry one item from the kitchen to the dinner table, rather than several.

Instead of serving each item in a separate bowl, or on a plate, everything goes into one beautifully presented container. You can use one compartment space for rice and the others for fish, meat and vegetable dishes. The compartments also act as guidelines for how much of each dish you need to serve. The boxes are made of three pieces: a bottom tray, a lid and an inner layer with compartments.

These rectangular boxes are stackable, and easy to transport from your kitchen to a dining room, or a patio. When it's time to do the washing up, you'll be amazed at how simple your Bento Box is to clean and put away.

Where to buy your Bento Box: go online or to a Japanese speciality store.

Your Japan Diet Small Shift

I am totally full and satisfied after a meal of several modest portions of healthy food enjoyed at a leisurely pace. I don't need to stuff myself.

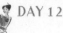

DAY 12

COLOUR YOUR LIFE WITH FRUIT AND VEGETABLES

Something beautiful is happening in the world of nutrition. A theory of 'superfoods' has been identified that is so powerful and so promising that nutritional authorities around the world are electrified by the concept. The reasons:

- It may help you lose weight by making you feel full with fewer calories.
- It may reduce your risk of having coronary heart disease, a heart attack or stroke.
- It may lower your blood pressure.
- It may reduce your risk of certain kinds of cancer.
- It may protect against major eye diseases – such as macular degeneration and cataract.
- It may protect against age-related decline in memory and thinking skills.
- It provides generous amounts of vitamins, fibre, minerals and phytonutrients.

The theory is not based on a new pill or a single nutrient, but on a simple, straightforward global insight that's as old as our grandparents' wisdom and as new as today's most cutting-edge clinical research:

The Superfoods Formula: to control your weight and fight chronic illness, eat a diet that is rich in many different fruits and vegetables.

If you want to get a dietitian or nutritional scientist worked up into a tizzy, just ask them about fruit and veg. They will start to practically swoon. They are totally besotted with the stuff. They believe that fruits and vegetables are extremely 'good' carbohydrates.

They are shouting it from the rooftops of their research laboratories and ivy-covered university sanctums: 'Eat more fruit and veg!'

Vegetables are a gift from nature. They have a million different flavours and textures. It doesn't have to mean eating carrot sticks all the time. People who really know how to enjoy vegetables eat lots of different vegetables and prepare them in different ways.

Vegetables, fruits and herbs contain the vitamins and minerals that we've known about for years, but they also carry phytochemicals, which contain the medicinal properties of foods. There are over 1,300 phytochemicals that have medicinal properties.

So when you eat your vegetables and fruits, and you eat a variety of them, you have a symphonic effect of all these beautiful nutrients helping your body stay strong; and recover from, repair and handle stress.

– Dr Ann Yelmokas McDermott, PhD
Research Scientist, Tufts University
USDA Human Nutrition Research Center

I must admit that I am flat-out addicted to vegetables. I was lucky to grow up at a time when vegetables were a superstar of the national food culture. Even today, after decades of Westernisation, vegetables still occupy a major portion of the Japanese diet. As we saw on the chart on pages 29–30, vegetable products are a much higher proportion of the Japanese diet compared with the UK, and Japanese people may eat a wider variety of veggies.

Japanese cuisine puts vegetables at the centre of a meal, transforming many different kinds of seasonal veggies into a series of colourful dishes bursting with flavours. You'd be amazed at the wide range of ways that vegetables are prepared in Japan – steamed, sautéed with subtle seasonings, simmered in delicious broth, dressed in mild vinaigrette, dressed in miso-based barbecue-like sauce. Often, several vegetables are mixed into one course, creating endless variations so you're never bored. I often make a couple of different vegetable dishes for one meal, each one with different vegetables, flavours and textures. Here's an example of how you can work five mouth-watering veggie dishes into a single meal:

Sample Menu: Five Vegetable Dishes in One Meal

Vegetable Dish	Colour	Method	Texture	Flavour	Recipe Page
Asparagus Salad with White Sesame Dressing	Bright dark green	Boil	Crisp, tender	Sweet	184
Beetroot Leaves Salad with Lemon Dressing	Red-green	Boil	Soft, not mushy	Citrusy	187
Kinpira Carrots with Hot Chilli Peppers	Orange	Sautée	Crisp, tender	Slightly Spicy hot	192
Radish Salad	White-green	Raw	Crisp, tender	Mildly Sour	184
Steamed Sweet Potatoes	Purple-yellow	Steam	Soft, chunky	Naturally sweet	216

I once heard that Westerners can regard eating vegetables as a punishment, dating from childhood when they were scolded crossly to 'eat your vegetables!' To me, veggies can be a scandalous pleasure. I don't have time to prepare fresh veggies every night, but when I do, I find the prepping and cooking to be therapeutic, almost like an instant meditation in your own kitchen! Washing, chopping, piling up cut vegetables in a colander feels wonderful. I take joy in the sound of water running out of the tap. I love the feel of cool water on my arms as I rinse the vegetables under running water. I like the splashes of water hitting against the vegetables in the sink.

The colours of fresh vegetables are magnificent, aren't they? The rich purple of aubergine, the stunning orange and red of peppers, the forest greens of broccoli and spinach. I love fresh herbs, too, such as coriander (*Coriandrum sativum*), also known as cilantro or Chinese parsley. When I snap a rubber band from around the stems and spread them out, the intoxicating aroma bursts out. I swish the bunch around in the sink and the leaves are drenched with sparkling water droplets. The bright green gets brighter. I break off a young jagged leaf from a sprig with my fingers. It looks and smells absolutely gorgeous.

Such a moment fills me with peace and happiness. I stand still. Gazing on the mounds of shiny colourful veggies in several colanders, 'What a miracle,' I murmur in my mind.

> *Fruit and vegetables are likely to reduce the risk of many cancers, especially those of the digestive system. These foods are high in many important nutrients and many of them are an excellent source of fibre. Cancer Research UK recommends eating at least five different portions of fruit and vegetables a day.*
>
> – Ed Yong
> Senior Health Information Officer
> Cancer Research UK

How can vegetables and fruits help you lose weight?

They can help you feel full on fewer calories, according to a widely respected theory of diet and nutrition called 'energy density' or 'calorie density'. This theory has been popularised by Dr Barbara Rolls, chair of the nutrition department at Penn State University. According to Dr Rolls, 'Fruits and vegetables really are key players in determining weight status.'

The calorie-density theory says that if you eat *more* 'low-calorie-dense' foods and *fewer* 'high-calorie-dense' foods, you will more effectively reach satiety, or fullness, and eat fewer calories overall.

- Low-calorie-dense foods and dishes include fruits, vegetables, low-fat milk, cooked grains, lean meats, poultry, fish, beans, broth-based soups, stews, pasta with vegetables and fruit-based desserts. You should eat more of them.
- High-calorie-dense foods include crackers, crisps, chocolates, pretzels, biscuits and butter. You should eat less of them.

The secret ingredient, according to this approach, is water, which dilutes the amount of calories in a given portion of food. 'Surprisingly, foods with a high water content have a big (positive) impact on satiety,' wrote Dr Rolls and Robert Barnett in their book *The Volumetrics Weight-Control Plan*. Of fruits and vegetables, they wrote: 'These carbohydrate-containing foods are truly extraordinary. You can eat virtually as much as you want of many of these and you'll wind up consuming fewer calories.'

Here's the mysterious thing about fruit and vegetables – we know they contain health-promoting substances, but we don't yet know much about how they work. 'Many people who know a little about phytochemicals (plant compounds that can support health) are waiting to hear about the one compound which, taken in large doses, will cure whatever ails them,' explained registered dietitian Karen Collins. 'Is it lycopene, beta carotene, or resveratrol? In fact, research seems to indicate that phytochemicals work together to boost our immune system. So you benefit by eating a great variety of plant foods containing a great variety of phytochemicals.'

In other words, the beneficial substances in fruit and veg seem to work in teams and highly complex patterns, so don't get too caught up in a single phytochemical or a list of only 'top 10 super-vegetables'. 'It is likely,' wrote epidemiologist Dr Lyn Steffen, of the University of Minnesota School of Public Health, in the January 2006 issue of *The Lancet,* 'that the combination of nutrients and compounds in foods has greater health benefits than the individual nutrient alone.' The bottom line, says the FSA, is 'we need to eat a variety of fruit and veg to make sure we get all the important nutrients we need'.

Population studies show that people who include plenty of fruit and vegetables in their diet tend to suffer less from a range of chronic diseases – such as heart disease, diabetes and certain kinds of cancers. Not only have vegetables got this whole range of nutrients and phytochemicals but they're also a great source of fibre. And we know that fibre not only helps with gut health but can help control things like cholesterol and might have a role to play with certain types of cancer.

– Dr Frankie Phillips, RD
British Dietetic Association

Tips for Super-charging your Fruit and Veg Lifestyle

The FSA urges us to 'eat a wide variety of fruit and vegetables and aim for at least five portions a day'. Unfortunately, only one in seven Britons is hitting that target and the average person eats about half the recommended amount. As a general guide, a 'portion' means 80 g, or any of these:

- 1 apple, banana, pear, orange or other similar-sized fruit
- 2 plums or similar-sized fruit
- ½ a grapefruit or avocado

- 1 slice of large fruit, such as melon or pineapple
- 3 heaped tablespoons of vegetables (raw, cooked, frozen or tinned)
- 3 heaped tablespoons of beans and pulses (however much you eat, beans and pulses count as a maximum of one portion a day)
- 3 heaped tablespoons of fruit salad (fresh or tinned in fruit juice) or stewed fruit
- 1 heaped tablespoon of dried fruit (such as raisins and apricots)
- 1 handful of grapes, cherries or berries
- a dessert bowl of salad
- a glass (150ml) of fruit juice (however much you drink, fruit juice counts as a maximum of one portion a day)

Fruit and veg should make up a third of the food you eat. Aim to eat at least five portions of fruit and veg every day. These can be fresh, frozen, tinned, dried or cooked, and a glass of fruit juice can also make up one of your portions each day. Remember potatoes are counted as a starchy food, not as portions of fruit and veg.

But it is important not to get hung up on portion sizes. If you make sure at least a third of your meals is made up by a variety of vegetables and you eat some fruit for pudding and at other times in the day, you'll easily reach your recommended amount.

All fruit and veg is nutritious, whether it's fresh, frozen or tinned, as long as it has little or no added salt or sugar.

Go organic, if you prefer. While there's no clear proof yet that organic is nutritionally superior, you may find, as I do, that organic produce tastes better, or is more in line with your personal philosophy.

Stock up your kitchen with vegetables and fruit – fresh produce from a farmers' market or supermarket, and tinned and frozen for short-cuts and emergencies. When you have a craving for a packet of biscuits, open the larder and reach for a tin of peaches.

Fruit and Vegetable Power-tips

Here are some ideas for boosting the amount of fruit and veg in your life. They include some of my tips together with suggestions from the Food Standards Agency (FSA), the National Institutes of Health (NIH) and the American Institute for Cancer Research (AICR):

- If you're not used to a veggie-intense lifestyle, phase extra veg in gradually over a period of a few weeks, to give your body time to adjust.
- Think of vegetables as the star of your meal, not just a side dish.
- Re-balance your plate to over two-thirds vegetables and less than one-third meat. You will feel full and satisfied, consume fewer calories and take in a richer variety of nutrients.
- If you currently eat only one or two different vegetables a day, add an extra serving at lunch and another at dinner.
- Think variety, variety, variety. In 2005, the *Wall Street Journal* featured their list of the 'ten top-rated nutritious fruits and vegetables'. These were spinach, romaine lettuce, broccoli, tomatoes, red and green peppers, cantaloupe, tangerines, blueberries, apricots and raspberries. Have you had any of these lately? If not, pick some up on your next trip to the market.
- Colourise your vegetable attitude: eat the whole spectrum of colours from all five vegetable subgroups – dark green, orange, legumes, starchy vegetables and other vegetables. Different-coloured vegetables provide different nutrients. Choose dark, leafy greens such as kale, spinach and mustard greens, and reds and oranges such as carrots, sweet potatoes, red peppers and tomatoes.
- Try gently steaming your vegetables, which is a very nutritious style of cooking. Use your electric steamer, or a cooker-top steamer, or try a bag of microwaveable steam fresh veggies.
- When you boil vegetables, be careful not to overcook them and use as little water as possible.
- Lightly season vegetables with herbs, lemon juice or sesame seeds instead of drenching them in butter, mayonnaise, creamy sauces and/or oily dressings.
- Include vegetables for breakfast. It's not such a radical idea –

you're already familiar with beans, mushrooms and tomatoes in your fry-up or bubble and squeak.

- Add vegetables or pulses to your curry, casserole or stir-fry. The term 'pulses' includes beans, lentils and peas. They are a low-fat source of protein, fibre, vitamins and minerals and count as a portion of fruit and veg. Pulses also count as a starchy food and add fibre to your meal. Three heaped tablespoons of pulses equals one portion.
- At your evening meal, serve at least two types of vegetables with your fish, chicken or meat.
- Include two or more vegetarian meals each week.
- At lunch, try a bowl of salad, have a banana sandwich or have some fruit salad.
- At breakfast, add a handful of dried fruit, blueberries and/or bananas to your cold or hot whole-grain cereal, eat half a grapefruit or an apple, or drink a glass of fruit juice. Choose fresh or tinned fruit more often than fruit juice. Fruit juice has little or no fibre.
- Use fruits or other foods low in saturated fat, trans fat, cholesterol, sodium, sugar and calories as desserts and snacks. Dried fruits are a good choice to carry with you or to have ready in the car.
- For a snack, reach for an apple, banana, dried fruit – or a vegetable such as sweet potato or carrot sticks.
- Eat a medium apple instead of four shortbread biscuits. You'll save 80 calories.
- Try to avoid adding sugar or syrupy extras to fruit, such as stewed apples.

Your Japan Diet Small Shift

I believe a diet rich in a wide variety of all fruit and veg is the real 'Superfood'.

DAY 13

HAVE A JAPAN-STYLE VEGETABLE MOMENT

On a recent summer day on the bucolic campus of Stanford University Medical School in California, a nutritional scientist, Christopher Gardner, took time off from his research to talk about a tasty subject, and one of his favourite dishes, stir-fried vegetables.

Gardner specialises in the role of nutrition and preventive medicine. He has published papers on soya and garlic; plant-based diets and phytochemicals; and cardiovascular disease and cancer prevention.

But when you hear the passion in Gardner's voice when he speaks of cooking and ingredients and colours and flavours, you get the feeling that maybe he's really in the business as much for the food as for the science. He said:

> If you look at the Japanese diet, the Mediterranean diet or the DASH (Dietary Approaches to Stop Hypertension) diet, there's a common theme: they are plant-based and nutrient-dense.
>
> Look at what Asians put in their stir-fries. The typical Japanese meal is *flavored* with strips of fish or chicken or beef. It's not a 12 oz porterhouse steak. There's rice, herbs that make it smell great and taste great, they've got water chestnuts and mange tout and mung sprouts, pak choi, mustard greens, just a wonderful variety of colours and flavours.

If you add it up, there are the classic vitamins, nutrients, phytochemicals and isoflavones.

It's not just what you should avoid, it's what you should include in your diet. You should include the nutrient-dense foods, of which you will find a lot in a Japanese diet. They're in vegetables, they're in beans, they're in wholegrains.

If you look at the emerging literature, you never find these positive factors in cheese or chicken or beef, they always seem to be coming, or at least 99 per cent of them, from the plant-based sources.

It's almost like 'who cares what the optimal amount is' – when you eat all those foods, you get them!

Why don't we take a quick food holiday together? For dinner tonight, let's make some Japan-style stir-fried vegetables. Go to the market and pick four or five beautiful-looking vegetables. Make sure they are fresh and seasonal.

Pick different colours, textures and flavours. For example, green peppers, sweet potatoes, yellow onions, carrots and broccoli. Chop them into bite sizes. Cut them into fairly uniform sizes so they cook at the same speed.

Heat 1 tbsp of rapeseed oil in a large frying pan or wok. Add the vegetables to the frying pan, in order of hardness, and stir-fry them at medium-high heat for 5 to 10 minutes.

Don't crowd the pan, or the vegetables will release too much liquid and become mushy. If you don't have enough space in the pan for all the veggies, cook them in batches and combine them at the end.

The beauty of this basic 'mini-recipe' is that you change your vegetable selection to create a different dish each time.

Write down what you taste and how you feel as you eat the veggies:

_____

_____

_____

Write down how you feel 10 minutes after the meal:

_____

_____

_____

Write down how you feel a few hours after the meal:

_____

_____

_____

Japan Diet vegetable showcase

Sweet potato

A deliciously complex carbohydrate food, it's been called 'the trendiest vegetable in Britain', and its sales are said to be growing faster than any other veg. A leading consumer group, the Center for Science in the Public Interest, calls them 'a nutritional All–Star: one of the best vegetables you can eat and 'loaded with carotenoids, vitamin C, potassium and fibre'.

It is the sweet potato, the lightly sugary-tasting vegetable that is loved by taste buds, celebrated by chefs such as Antony Worrall Thompson, Brian Turner and Hugh Fearnley-Whittingstall and praised by dietitians. 'Due to their antioxidant and fibre content, they are protective against heart disease and cancer,' said registered dietitian Cynthia Sass. 'The high levels of phytochemicals and beta-carotene also help protect the eye from disorders like macular degeneration.'

Tesco produce buyer Tarik Abdel-Hady told the *Daily Mail* in May 2006 that 'apart from its unique sweet and nutty taste much of the sweet potato's popularity stems from it being delicious and filling but low in fat making it a dieter's dream.' He praised the veg as 'extremely versatile' and 'easy and quick to prepare'.

Japanese people love sweet potatoes. When I was growing up in Japan, they were such a big part of the diet that sweet potato wagons would come to our neighbourhood of Tokyo offering the vegetable as an afternoon snack.

You should welcome the sweet potato into your home, as one of the tastiest and most nutritious members of the pantheon of veggies.

Sweet potato tips:

- Look for firm sweet potatoes with smooth skins and no soft spots.
- Don't put them in the refrigerator, place them in a dry, cool and dark spot.
- Bake a sweet potato in the oven for about 1 hour and 45 minutes at 150°C/Gas Mark 2. Place in a dish and/or wrap in aluminium foil since caramelisation of the sugars can be released and mess up your oven.
- Or microwave a sweet potato with the skin on for about 6 minutes on full power (about 1,000 watt microwave) followed immediately by wrapping in aluminium foil for two minutes once out of the microwave.
- Or cut into bite-size pieces and steam them, for 10 minutes or until cooked through.
- Don't put sugary toppings on them, they're naturally sweet already.

Sea vegetables, a gift from the ocean

If sweet potatoes are the UK's 'It food' of the moment, then sea vegetables, less glamorously known as seaweed, are hot on their heels. This gently crunchy, sometimes smoky and always hearty treat is shedding its shyness and stepping out into the recipes of top chefs and home cooks alike. In BBC2's Great British Menu competition in 2005, chef Richard Corrigan proposed green sea lettuce as part of his perfect menu for the Queen's 80th-birthday banquet. At London's Paternoster Square Chop House, head chef Peter Weeden served it with seafood alongside traditional British dishes, and he has been reported to whip up vegetarian bubble and squeak made with Welsh-inspired seaweed-based laverbread.

In Japan, sea vegetables are integral to the diet. So much so that they are everywhere, as a garnish, a condiment and as a key ingredient of dashi cooking stock (see page 168).

So, what is there to love about seaweed? First, there's the taste. If you love sushi, then you already love the flavourful nori seaweed that it's wrapped in. There are also nutritional reasons to consider when incorporating moderate amounts of seaweed into your diet. Seaweed, particularly the brown varieties such as wakame and kombu, said research toxicologist Christine Skibola, PhD, of the University of California School of Public Health, 'may be one of the major cancer-protecting components of the Japanese diet'.

Besides being high in fibre, B vitamins and the minerals magnesium, calcium and iodine, Dr Skibola said that seaweed contains high levels of bioactive compounds 'that have been associated with antioxidant, anti-inflammatory and antiviral activity'.

However, she warns that 'some can also contain high levels of iodine that could be deleterious to individuals sensitive to iodine'. But beyond that, Dr Skibola concludes, 'We're starting to see now that seaweed may have a lot of health benefits.'

I think a simple way to bring these mineral-rich treasures from the sea into your meals is to introduce them first as condiments. Get a container of shredded nori sea vegetables at a Japanese grocery store and use it in place of the salt shaker on your dining table. Sprinkle a few shreds over rice, or put some into your miso soup or stir-fry. Mix a small quantity of wakame sea vegetables into salads and stir-fries.

When you dine out at a Japanese restaurant, or have a Japanese takeaway, explore small dishes that include sea vegetables, to see which ones you like best, and gradually introduce them to your dining table.

Your Japan Diet Small Shift

I believe vegetables are not a punishment.
They are not boring.
They are sexy and delicious.
Vegetables are a tempting and scandalous nutritional pleasure.

DAY 14

SWIM IN THE GOOD FATS – WITH FISH

A man in Pennsylvania has uncovered a mystery about Japan. 'There's something about the Japanese diet and lifestyle that seems to be unique,' he said, and it may help protect Japanese people against coronary heart disease, one of the world's biggest killers.

It is a paradox, something he can't exactly figure out. But he has an interesting theory and it involves the power of fish. Dr Lewis Kuller is an elder statesman in the field of epidemiology, the study of populations and public health. He has studied medicine for nearly 50 years, he is a doctor of medicine and a University Professor of Public Health at the University of Pittsburgh Graduate School of Public Health. He has published over 500 articles in medical journals.

Kuller and his colleagues in Japan have been studying patterns of diet and disease among Japanese people and comparing them to populations elsewhere in the world. And they've noticed something that he finds absolutely fascinating.

According to Dr Kuller, among Japanese men who are in their 40s and 50s today, there has been a shift towards more Western lifestyles and eating habits. They are eating more saturated fat, meat and cheese than their elders did. They are very heavy smokers. They have hypertension. They are becoming less physically active. They eat lots of eggs and have one of the highest cholesterol intakes in the world.

We should be seeing a sharp rise in the increase in coronary heart disease among Japanese, said Dr Kuller. There should be an epidemic of heart attacks in Japan. You'd expect the rates to be going 'off the scale'. But they're not. In fact, they're not moving much at all. Dr Kuller reports: 'There's very little evidence of an increase in coronary heart disease incidence or mortality in the Japanese population, especially in the fairly young Japanese population. That to me is an important unexplained paradox.'

It's not a genetic effect unique to Asians, he reasons, because 'we've studied the Japanese in America, Brazil and Hawaii, and their rates are much higher' than those in Japan. Also the Chinese are seeing increasing rates of coronary heart disease, and rates are going up in Taiwan, South Korea and Singapore as well.

'It may well be that something in the [Japanese] diet is protective, which we could add to our diet,' he speculates. He can't prove it, but if he had to place a bet today, Kuller said he'd wager that the answer to the paradox is that the Japanese enjoy 'an extraordinarily high intake of omega-3 fatty acids from fish'.

The Japan I grew up in was truly a fish-crazed nation and it still is today. The food culture is intensely focused on celebrating fish in the daily diet, in an enormous range of varieties and cooking styles. Japanese are fish-eating champions of the world, not only beating the UK and USA by a wide margin, but, according to Dr Kuller, 'they eat a lot more fish than the Chinese' and 'about twice as much as the Koreans'.

His hypothesis is that it's the very high intake of omega-3s in the Japanese diet that is heart-protective and a key factor contributing towards the high longevity of the Japanese people.

What does it mean for us in the West? 'Keeping saturated fat as low as possible and dramatically increasing the amount of omega-3 fatty acids in the diet might have very big benefits,' said Kuller, 'and we need to find that out.'

As with so much in the diet and nutrition world, the research on fish is not iron-clad. Many studies have suggested health benefits for oily fish, mainly in protecting the heart. But a 2006 review paper in the *British Medical Journal* found little firm evidence of such benefits, leading Joe Schwarcz, Professor of Chemistry at McGill

University, to write that 'it is clear that we cannot swallow all the hype about the supposed miraculous properties of omega-3 fats hook, line and sinker'. He speculated, 'Maybe the benefits of fish are not in what they contain, but in what they displace from the diet. Better to eat fish than hamburgers or trans fat laden fries.'

But if Dr Kuller is right about the benefits that Japanese people enjoy from fish, his theory would dovetail with a consensus that is emerging throughout the nutritional world: *fat, of the right type and in the proper balance, is good.* More specifically, 'good fats' like the omega-3s in fish can be an important component of a healthy diet.

As you probably know by now, the consensus is that there are 'good fats and bad fats'. Some fats harm our heart and health – while others help them.

Bad fats: eat less

* *Saturated fat* is found in whole milk, ice cream, cheese, butter and red meat, among other foods. Eat less saturated fat, because it increases the risk of heart disease.
  * This is A LOT of fat:
    20 g fat or more per 100 g
    5 g saturates or more per 100 g
  * This is A LITTLE fat – try to choose these:
    3 g fat or less per 100 g
    1 g saturates or less per 100 g

If the amount of total fat is between 3 g and 20 g per 100 g, this is a moderate amount of total fat. Between 1 g and 5 g of saturates is a moderate amount of saturated fat.

* *Trans fat* can be found in fast food, chips, doughnuts, and commercially baked products, such as biscuits, margarines and hydrogenated vegetable oils. Eat much less trans fat, because it increases the risk of heart disease. The good news is that many food companies are already reducing the volume of trans fats.

Good fats: eat more

- *Monounsaturated fat* is found in rapeseed oil (non-hydrogenated is best), olive oil, olives, peanut oil, avocados and many nuts.
- *Polyunsaturated fat* is found in vegetable oils such as soya oil (non-hydrogenated is best), legumes including soya beans and soya products – and oily fish.

Oily fish is hailed as one of the best ways to get omega-3s into your diet. In 2002, the World Health Organization found that 'most . . . population studies have shown that fish consumption is associated with a reduced risk of coronary heart disease'. In 2005, a 'generic health claim' was approved in the UK that 'eating 3 g weekly, or 0.45 g daily, long-chain omega-3 polyunsaturated fatty acids, as part of a healthy lifestyle, helps maintain heart health'.

One of the biggest supporters of fish these days is the Food Standards Agency. Take a look at what the FSA has been telling us:

- Most of us should be eating more fish – aim for at least two portions a week, including a portion of oily fish, which is high in omega-3s.
- Oily fish includes salmon, sardines, herring and mackerel.
- You can choose from fresh, frozen or tinned – but remember that tinned and smoked fish can be high in salt.
- Women of childbearing age should limit their intake to a maximum of two portions of oily fish a week (a portion is about 140 g/5 oz). For all other adults the recommended weekly maximum is four portions.
- Anyone who regularly eats a lot of fish should choose as wide a variety as possible.
- White fish such as cod, haddock, plaice and whiting are very low in fat. Therefore, although they do contain some omega-3 fatty acids, it is at much lower levels than oily fish.
- Fish is an excellent source of protein and contains essential vitamins and minerals, such as selenium and iodine. Oily fish

(such as salmon, eel, fresh tuna and pilchards) is a good
source of vitamins A and D, too.

• Fish such as whitebait, tinned sardines, pilchards and salmon
  – where you also eat the bones – are also good sources of
  calcium and phosphorus, which help make our bones
  stronger.

There has been controversy and some confusion over the safety of
fish, owing to fears over contaminants that some species may
contain such as mercury and polychlorinated biphenyls (PCBs:
industrial by-products, now banned, that still persist in the
environment). The most problematic fish are long-lived predatory
species, such as marlin, shark and swordfish. They are at the top
of the food chain and so may accumulate large amounts of
contaminants from the fish they prey on. Some researchers have
also raised concerns over what they see as high levels of PCBs
found in farmed salmon, from the fish oil and fish meal they are
fed on.

The FSA, on the other hand, has dismissed these claims as
exaggerated, declaring that the health benefits for oily fish 'clearly
outweigh the possible risks'. The advantages of eating fish 'are likely
to be at least 100-fold greater than the estimates of harm, which
may not exist at all,' argued Walter Willett, professor of nutrition at
the Harvard School of Public Health.

There are, however, clear consumption guidelines for different
fish depending on your age, sex and 'lifestage', which the FSA has
summarised in this chart:

Oily fish: who should eat what?
Food Standards Agency

	Fertile/pregnant women	Breastfeeding women
Oily fish	Up to 2 portions a week	Up to 2 portions a week
White fish	No limit	No limit
Tinned tuna**	Up to 4 medium-size tins	No limit on tinned
Marlin, shark, swordfish	Do not eat	Up to 1 portion a week

	Infertile women	Men
Oily fish	Up to 4 portions a week	Up to 4 portions a week
White fish	No limit	No limit
Tinned tuna**	No limit on tinned	No limit on tinned
Marlin, shark, swordfish	Up to 1 portion a week	Up to 1 portion a week

*A portion = 140 g (5 oz)
** Only fresh tuna counts as oily fish, as most of the natural oils are lost from tinned tuna during the canning process.

What's an oily fish?

Oily/fatty fish

Anchovies	Jack fish	Salmon
Bloater	Katla	Sardines
Cacha	Kipper	Sprats
Carp	Mackerel	Swordfish
Eel	Orange roughy	Trout
Herring	Pangas	Tuna (fresh only)
Hilsa	Pilchards	Whitebait

Naomi's Top Five Tips for Enjoying More Fish in Your Life

Tinned salmon, herring, mackerel and sardines are fabulous ways to enjoy oily fish regularly. They are super-convenient. They are as nutritious as fresh. And the skin and soft bones in tinned salmon are completely edible and good for you, too.

1. Look for tinned fish with less sodium.
2. Choose poached, baked, steamed or grilled fish instead of fried. Fried fish is much higher in fat, especially when deep-fried in batter.
3. Instead of mayonnaise, tartar sauce, hollandaise sauce, or butter, try seasoning fish with:

   - Lemon juice.
   - Chopped herbs.
   - Traditional Japanese-style flavourings such as a small mound of grated radish and a few drops of low-sodium soy sauce, or citrus juice flavoured soy sauce.
   - A dash of teriyaki sauce.
   - Some low-sodium mustard.
   - Creamy tofu sauce (see recipe page 171).

4. Have a piece of fresh or tinned fish with your breakfast. It doesn't have to only be kippers!
5. For information on the environmental sustainability and safety of different fish, as well as handy 'fish lists' you can use when you go shopping, check out the 'resources' section at the end of this book.

Your Japan Diet Small Shift

I'm going to eat more fish in my diet, especially oily fish like salmon, sardines, herring and mackerel.

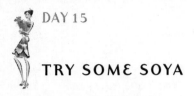

DAY 15

TRY SOME SOYA

Not long ago I was in Tokyo, having lunch with my sister Miki and her family at one of our favourite spots, a restaurant called Umenohana, which means Plum Blossoms.

This is a nation-wide, family-style chain that strikes a perfect balance of elegance and comfort. There is no communal main dining room. Instead every party is escorted to an individual dining room. Umenohana is unusual because the entire restaurant is dedicated to celebrating a single food, tofu, a delicacy made from soaked and pressed soya beans. The meal is served 'kaiseki style', which means in a relaxed procession of little dishes.

• • • • •

The waitress presents us with dishes of tofu shumai dumpling, simmered tofu and grilled tofu with sweet miso dressing, along with cups of steamed tofu-egg custard called *chawan mushi*. After these courses, she simmers some soya milk in a square pan in the middle of the table, until it forms a thin vanilla-yellow tofu skin, called 'yuba'. Yuba is a Kyoto-speciality and perhaps more of a delicacy than tofu and is transformed into many exquisite dishes.

The waitress carefully lifts it up, places it in a bowl with dipping sauce and hands the bowl to us to enjoy while it is still hot. Then into the room come plates of fried shrimp wrapped in yuba, tofu chunks on hot grilling stones, bowls of clear soup with yuba, steamed rice, tiny pickled vegetables, followed by custard pudding, yes, made of tofu, and finally – as always – green tea.

What's remarkable about this experience is the amazing variety of sensations that the restaurant can squeeze out of one food theme. The tofu dishes have so many succulent flavours, colourful shades and intriguing textures: warm or cool, firm-and-meaty, silken-smooth, custardy-sweet.

• • • • •

Japan has a passion for soya that's been going on for over a thousand years, and in the course of an average day you can easily have soya at every meal. You could have miso soup for breakfast, some tofu with your lunch, some edamame beans as a beer snack with your friends after work, and some soy sauce and natto (fermented soya beans) with your dinner.

You can see how soya has worked its way into the Japanese diet, as well as the Chinese and Korean diets, as a regular source of protein, by taking a look at these 2003 calorie supply estimates below from the United Nations. Some people mistakenly believe that Asian countries consume massive amounts of soya products, but you can see that it still takes a minority position, although intake is much higher than the UK and USA:

Daily Protein Per Person, in Grams

	Meat	Fish	Soya beans
Japan	14.0	23.4	8.7
Korea	15.8	16.2	6.2
China	17.5	5.9	3.4
UK	29.4	5.7	0.02
US	40.9	4.7	0.02

Many nutritional experts are fans of soya as a source of non-animal protein, and they tend to rank the different kinds of soya product according to how close they are to the original bean. Edamame soya beans are placed on top, with semi-processed tofu and miso products next, and highly processed types such as soy sauce and soya chips placed last.

One drawback of tofu is that it loses much of its fibre during processing. However, one advantage, according to Dr Barbara Rolls, chair of the Penn State University nutrition department, is that tofu is 'low-calorie dense', meaning it fills you up and satisfies you more effectively than meat or cheese, both of which by comparison are higher in calorie density. I often use tofu instead of meat for this reason.

Tofu is filling and satisfying and absorbs the delicious juicy flavours of whatever I cook it in. I can choose to buy any one of several different textures – from silken to very firm. I chop tofu into my stir-fries, or into my morning miso soup, or as a cool side dish. The best part: tofu is a good protein source and yet, unlike red meat, has virtually no saturated fat.

Japan Diet fashion spotlight: edamame, the chic green treat

Smaller than a lima bean, edamame (eh-dah-MAH-meh) are immature soya beans that can be served in their pods or shelled. They're a trendy food that fit perfectly into a mostly plant-based diet that, as we have seen, research suggests reduces the risk of cancer and other diseases. You can find fresh or frozen edamame soya beans at Oriental or Japanese markets and some grocery stores.

Edamame must be cooked before serving. If the edamame soya beans you buy are uncooked, boil them in water for 7 to 8 minutes until tender.

In Japan and China, edamame soya beans are popular as snacks served in the shell. You need to pop the beans out before eating them.

Shelled edamame can be added to salads, stir-fries and mixed vegetable side dishes. Or you can add them to soups during the last 10 minutes of simmering. They replace peas beautifully in casseroles.

Although edamame soya beans look like vegetables and have a buttery, nutty flavour similar to baby lima beans, they make a healthy meat substitute.

A serving of cooked beans contains 11 g of protein and 4 g of fibre. Small portions of them are very satisfying.

Soya, regrettably, has been over-hyped in the media and by some experts. Many people, for example, point to the low breast cancer rates among women in Japan and jump to the conclusion that the reason is because soya is protective against this disease.

But that cause and effect has never been clearly proven, and the low Japanese breast cancer rates could just as well be the result of something else that is or isn't in the diet, for example less saturated fat from meat. Soya has likewise often been promoted as a solution to menopausal hot flushes, but in October 2005, the US Agency for Healthcare Research and Quality called most of the research in this area to be 'inconclusive' and of 'poor quality'.

'I think overall the research on soya is really uncompelling,' declared the straight-talking Professor Marion Nestle, chair of the New York University Nutrition Department, in an interview given to the *San Francisco Chronicle* last year. 'What the data shows is that if there is harm from soya, it is very small; and if there are benefits, they are also very small. That means the data revolves around zero.'

Here is how Ed Yong, Senior Health Information Officer of Cancer Research UK, summed up the evidence on soya and cancer: 'Scientists are still uncertain about how eating soya products can affect the risk of cancer. Some studies have linked eating soya products, such as tofu, soya milk or miso, to reduced risk of breast, prostate and bowel cancer. This may be one reason why Asian people have lower risks of these cancers compared with Western people, but these differences may be due to other factors.' He concluded that 'clinical trials are needed to say for sure if soya affects the risk of cancer' either positively or negatively.

The possible link between soya and reduced breast-cancer risk got something of a boost in a study published in the 5 April 2006 issue of *The Journal of the National Cancer Institute* (JNCI), which analysed data from 18 previously published studies. The study concluded that among healthy women, soya consumption was associated with a small but statistically significant reduction in breast-cancer risk.

According to Karen Collins, Registered Dietitian and nutrition advisor to the American Institute for Cancer Research, 'The JNCI study supports the notion that soya has a place as one component of a cancer-protective diet high in a variety of plant foods and low in meat and dairy products. It's no miracle food, but it offers a healthy and versatile alternative to meat that can add variety to meals.'

Soya has also been promoted as a heart protector, because of its possible effect of lowering LDL 'bad' cholesterol. In the UK, a health claim was approved in 2002 that read: 'The inclusion of at least 25 g soya protein per day as part of a diet low in saturated fat can help reduce blood cholesterol.' A similar statement approved by the US Food and Drug Administration in 1999 allowed companies to claim that foods containing soya protein 'may reduce the risk of heart disease'.

The American Heart Association concluded in early 2006, however, that soya has in fact a negligible effect on cholesterol and is not likely to prevent heart disease, but added that soya products were still a healthy substitute for animal protein sources that are high in saturated fat, as well as providing polyunsaturated fat, fibre, vitamins and minerals.

'Soya is a good substitute for animal protein and, of the plant sources, soya is probably the best,' said global obesity expert and clinical nutritionist Dr Benjamin Caballero, MD, of the Johns Hopkins Bloomberg School of Public Health. The reason, he reports, is 'most other plant sources of protein are either limited in some essential amino acids or they don't have good digestibility'.

I love moderate amounts of soya-based foods, edamame and tofu in particular, not only because of what I am taking into my body, but also what I am not. When I eat tofu instead of fatty meat, I am consuming less saturated fat in my diet.

That is the 'Soya lesson' of the Japanese diet – soya is not a miracle food, but in moderate amounts it can be a good high-protein replacement for less-healthy foods.

Naomi's Top Three Soya Tips

1. Pick up some frozen edamame at a Japanese market and boil some up as a snack or part of a meal.

2. Try firm, plain tofu as an alternative to meat. Slice some little squares into your soup, salad or stir-fry.

3. Talk to your doctor or dietitian about how you could include soya in your diet. Some experts see the moderate consumption patterns of soya in the Far East as a useful guide – for example, two or three servings of soya-based products a week. Some people are allergic to soya, so check with your GP or dietitian for more information.

Your Japan Diet Small Shift

I'm going to try some natural soya products like edamame and tofu in moderation as an alternative to foods high in saturated fat.

DAY 16

UNLEASH THE POWER OF RICE AND WHOLEGRAINS

The 'Shangri La' of Healthy Eating in Japan may lie on a narrow side street in Tokyo's fashionable Omotesando neighbourhood, in a sleek, tranquil restaurant called the Brown Rice Café.

Here, they've taken the nutritious foundations of the Japanese diet and pushed them to a delightful extreme. The stars of the show are vegetables in season, tofu, tea and wholegrain brown rice, the kind that Japanese people ate centuries ago before white rice became popular.

You can order the Brown Rice Pouch Set, a fried tofu pouch filled with brown rice, ratatouille and miso, or the Bean and Vegetable Curry, served with brown rice, salad and home-made pickles with spice.

To drink, how about a cup of brown rice green tea or a glass of freshly squeezed soya milk? For dessert, the choices include a moist Tofu Tart served with lemon sauce and soya cream, and a fruit cake made of organic dried fruit, sesame, buckwheat flour and, you guessed it – soya and brown rice.

The Brown Rice Café is right on the cutting edge of the wholegrains revolution, one of the hottest healthy trends in the diet and nutrition world. But you don't have to spend 14 hours flying to Tokyo to reap the benefits – it can take as little as 90 seconds in your kitchen – by popping a pouch of 90-second brown rice from the supermarket into your microwave.

It's no secret that rice is the bedrock of most Asian diets, especially in Japan, where it is served in its own little bowl with almost every meal cooked at home, often even at breakfast. Japanese have discovered a multitude of uses for rice, in wine, beer, cooking oil, crackers, vinegar, soup and noodles. Rice is a low-fat, complex carbohydrate that fills you up, gives you energy and leaves less room for unhealthy foods such as biscuits and pastries.

Brown rice, which was Japan's original ancient power food, is a great wholegrain, high-fibre choice and is filled with a tempting hearty and nutty flavour.

How is rice, especially brown rice, so healthy?

Rice, along with bread, cereals, pasta and potatoes, is a complex (or starchy) carbohydrate, and so is the foundation of a healthy diet. The FSA says complex carbs should make up about a third of our meals. And the agency urges us to choose wholegrain varieties, such as brown rice, whenever we can as they contain vitamins, minerals and fibre necessary for good health and can help with weight control.

Like fruit and veg, wholegrains are low-calorie-density and may help you stay fuller on fewer calories than higher-calorie-dense foods. There may be heart-healthy benefits to wholegrains, too. In the UK in 2002, a generic health claim was approved for wholegrain products that reads: 'People with a healthy heart tend to eat more wholegrain foods as part of a healthy lifestyle.' The claim applies to foods containing 51 per cent or more wholegrain ingredients by weight per serving. The term 'wholegrains' includes wheat, rice, maize and oats, and refers to minimally processed grains in which all three components – endosperm, germ and bran – are retained.

Spotlight on wholegrains
According to the British Dietetic Association:
- Wholegrains may help you maintain a healthy body weight.
- 95 per cent of adults don't eat enough wholegrains.
- Most of the cereal foods consumed in the UK are refined – and therefore not 'whole' grain.
- Wholegrains have up to 75 per cent more nutrients than refined cereals.
- Eating wholegrains as part of a healthy diet and lifestyle may also help reduce the risk of many common diseases, including heart disease, Type 2 diabetes and some forms of cancer of the digestive tract.

There are many different wholegrain choices you can enjoy:
- Meal accompaniments: brown rice, wholewheat pasta, whole barley, bulgur wheat (cracked wheat), quinoa, pearl barley.
- Breakfast cereals: whole oats including rolled oats and oatmeal, wholewheat cereals, wholegrain muesli and wholegrain cereal bars.
- Bread and crackers: wholemeal, granary, wheatgerm, multi-grain, seeded or mixed-grain bread, soya and linseed breads, wholewheat crackers and pitta; rye bread (pumpernickel), rye crispbread, wholegrain ricecakes and oatcakes.
- Flour: wholemeal flour, wheat germ, buckwheat flour, unrefined rye and barley flour, oatmeal and oat flour.

Personally, I enjoy all kinds of rice – especially medium- and short-grain brown rice, premium short-grain koshihikari white rice (this is the leading table rice in Japan and you can get it at a Japanese market or online), short-grain sushi rice and partially polished haiga-mai rice, which contains the nutritious rice germ, but not the bran. I find them all totally delicious, filling and perfect complements to any food and very often at least a co-star of my meals, all through the day. I have an electric rice cooker and most of the day you'll find it cooking, or switched on to the timer setting, ready to cook.

Japanese-style rice has a different taste from what you might be used to, and you could find it quite delightful. It's moister, a bit sweeter and slightly stickier (but not gummy) than long-grain varieties, which I personally think are a tad dry. Its subtle flavour is a perfect companion for all the other dishes you serve. And, because of its naturally wonderful flavour and texture, medium- or short-grain rice does not need butter or oil to cook. So you're not only eating healthy starchy food and grains, you are avoiding excess bad fats.

Supporters of the glycaemic index approach to nutrition say we should limit our consumption of white rice because they believe it spikes our blood glucose levels too quickly and too sharply, thereby raising our risk of obesity. This opinion has many distinguished supporters, including Dr Walter Willett at the Harvard University School of Public Health, who says we should use white rice sparingly, along with red meat, butter, white bread, white pasta, potatoes, fizzy drinks and sweets. And a Japanese study published last year based on questionnaires of 1,354 rural Japanese female farmers found a connection between white rice consumption, glycaemic load and higher body mass index.

The anti-white-rice people may have a perfectly valid point, but personally I'm not totally convinced yet. Back in 1999, in fact, a team of Japanese researchers published a paper arguing that Japanese-style short-grain white rice should *not* be classified as high GI. Also, the GI experts at the University of Sydney told us last year that while their latest tests found Japan-style short-grain white rice to be 'high GI', they ran tests on sushi samples made from salmon and white rice and found them to be 'low GI'.

I also find the opinion of this top nutritional expert to be really interesting:

Dr Benjamin Caballero is Clinical Nutritionist at the Johns Hopkins Bloomberg School of Public Health and Editor in Chief of the *Encyclopedia of Human Nutrition*. He explained:

If you take white rice by itself, it's a carbohydrate that is absorbed very quickly and tends to create higher blood sugar levels than would wild rice or unpolished brown rice. However, the consumption of rice with other components, with some condiment or vegetable, quickly changes the rate of absorption so it becomes a more progressive increase in blood sugar.

That's why it is so difficult to use the glycemic index to rate foods, because it depends a lot on what else you eat. The GI is calculated for each food in the pure form. So if you mix two or three foods, the GI in terms of the blood sugar response will change completely.

Glycemic index is more useful in the management of diabetes and in controlling blood sugar in people who have glucose intolerance and are under the care of a dietitian, but for the general population it's more difficult to apply, because it changes so much in terms of the combinations of different foods and the preparation of different foods and how you cook it. It is an interesting concept but I think the practical application is still not there.

Rice is my bread and butter. Japanese-style rice is my soul food – and it can be yours, too.

It is warm, comforting, soothing and filling. When it is luxuriating in its own bowl it looks like a minimalist painting, yet when you chew it with other foods it somehow becomes dazzlingly complex.

When rice is cooked, the grains glisten in earthy brown or silvery white shades, exuding a steamy intoxicating aroma. A bonus point: since the short and medium rice grains gently stick together, it's easy to scoop up a mouthful with a pair of chopsticks. This is harder to do with long-grain rice.

I love brown rice not only for its flavour, but also because it has much more fibre and nutrients than white rice. I enjoy short-grain white rice as well, not only because it tastes exquisitely delicious and was a pillar of the diet I grew up with, but because I know it helps me fill up on healthy meals and leaves me almost no room to crave so-called junk foods.

That's the part I like the most.

Five Top Tips for Eating More Rice and Wholegrains

1. Have a bowl of brown rice with your meals rather than biscuits, white bread, or rolls. A bowl or two of naturally 'low-calorie-dense' rice, either brown or white, with your meal helps you fill up and stay satisfied, leaving less room for belly-busting desserts. Have a bite of rice to start your meal, move on to your other dishes and come back periodically for the rice. By rotating your tastes, the rice acts as a bridge between different foods, cleanly complementing and enhancing the flavours of the other foods. If you're a devotee of the glycaemic index approach, choose brown rice over white.

2. Take the instant brown rice shortcut: pick up a pouch of 90-second microwaveable brown rice, which you can get at most supermarkets. It's a great, ultra-fast way to welcome rice to your table with absolutely no fuss.

3. Cook and serve your rice without oil, salt or butter: the secret of Japan-style rice is minimalism – nothing is added to the saucepan, or to the cooked rice at the table. Short- and medium-grain rice is delicious cooked plain, with water. It's easy, but it does take time. See the recipes opposite.

4. Get a good electric rice cooker for super-convenience. This is really the best option to bring rice into your diet. An electric rice cooker makes perfect rice each time, with very little effort. All you have to do is to put the water and rice in the pot and press the 'on' button, just like brewing coffee in a coffee maker. No mess, little fuss. And most electric rice cookers

come with a timer and 'keep warm' functions, so you can have a hot and fluffy batch already cooked when you come home from work, or when you wake up in the morning.

5.   For more wholegrains, replace refined cereal foods with wholegrain versions. The British Dietetic Association advises us to look for the word 'whole' before the name of the cereal, such as whole oats and wholewheat pasta. It also advises us to opt for two or three servings of wholegrains a day.

FLUFFY JAPANESE SHORT- OR MEDIUM-GRAIN RICE (BROWN, WHITE OR HAIGA)

MAKES 750 g (1½ lb)

Cooker-top method

. . . .

370 g (13 oz) short- or medium-grain rice (brown, white or haiga)
570 ml (1 pint) cold water for white rice or haiga-mai; 680 ml (1¼ pints) for brown rice

. . . .

Wash the rice (unless you are using haiga-mai) by putting the grains in a medium bowl and adding cold water to cover. Swish the grains with your hand to remove the starch and then drain off the cloudy water by tilting the bowl and holding the rice in the bowl with a cupped palm. Repeat this process two or three more times, or until the water when agitated around the rice is almost clear. Drain the rice in a fine-mesh sieve. (Some brands of rice do not require washing: please read directions on the package.) To cook the rice, transfer the washed grains to a medium saucepan. Add the cold water and let the rice sit in the water 20 minutes to plump.

Cover the saucepan and bring the rice to the boil. Reduce the heat to low and gently simmer the rice for 15 minutes (longer for brown rice), or until all liquid is evaporated. Turn off the heat and let the rice sit, covered, for 10 minutes. When ready to serve, fluff the rice grains by gently turning them over with a wet wooden, or plastic, rice paddle.

Electric rice cooker method

··············
370 g (13 oz) short- or medium-grain rice (brown, white or haiga)
Cold water
··············

Wash the rice according to the instructions indicated above for the Stove-top Method. To cook the rice, transfer the washed grains to the cooking bowl of an electric rice cooker. Add enough cold water to the bowl, according to the machine's instructions, for 370 g of dry rice. Let the rice sit in the water 20 minutes to plump. Plug in the rice cooker and push the On or Start button. When the rice has finished cooking, let it rest undisturbed for 10 minutes (do not open the lid). When ready to serve, fluff the rice grains by gently turning them over with a wet wooden, or plastic, rice paddle.

Your Japan Diet Small Shift

I'm going to add some brown rice and other wholegrains to my diet.

DAY 17

BE GENTLE TO YOUR FOOD

One of the healthiest aspects of the Japanese diet is the cooking style. It is super-light, ultra-gentle – and simple in character. And sometimes food is not cooked at all.

Japanese cuisine uses delicious, healthy cooking stock, such as fish-and-sea-vegetable stock (dashi – see page 168), healthy oils such as rapeseed and healthy techniques such as simmering and steaming. Ingredients including vinegar, soy sauce and sake (rice wine) are added in modest amounts to complement the food's personality, not compete with it.

Japan-style cooking is also easier than you might think. Most of the cooking and preparation happens on the stove and on the worktop, and it happens relatively quickly. There is virtually no oven roasting, or baking for hours at a time.

You can adopt the healthiest lessons of Japan-style cooking almost instantly.

The mantra is minimalism: 'Less is more.' The great food writer M.F.K. Fisher calls it a style that says, 'Let simple seem like much, as long as it is fresh and beautiful.'

The style is expressed by what food historian Naomichi Ishige calls the 'fundamental philosophy of traditional Japanese cooking'. These are three interconnected ideas that can help you bring The Japan Diet into your life.

The first point, in Mr Ishige's words, is:

*'Food should be enjoyed as close as possible to its natural state,
with the minimum of artificial technique.'*

This idea is not too different from what the great French chef
Auguste Escoffier used to urge to his apprentices: 'Stay simple!
Cook simply!' A vivid Japanese illustration of this is *sashimi* (raw
fish), and other examples include the many lightly dressed Japanese
vegetable dishes. With few exceptions, very little animal fat is used
in Japanese cooking.

You can also see the 'close to nature' theme on gorgeous
display in the form of the tableware you are presented with at
a Japanese restaurant. Made of bamboo, unfinished wood,
ceramics and red and black lacquer, the vessels resemble objects
you might glimpse in a forest, such as a stone, a twig (chopsticks)
or an oak leaf.

The second foundation of Japanese food philosophy, declared
Mr Ishige, is a point often made by Japanese cooks:

*'The ability to select fresh ingredients and enhance natural flavour
is more important than cooking technique.'*

Isn't that an interesting idea? The challenge isn't 'how to cook' the
food, but how to *select it*.

Fresh ingredients are an obsession in Japanese food culture,
with both high street chefs and housewives relentlessly searching
for the fish and produce that are in season, or 'shun'. At my
mother's local grocery store, and any others in Japan, the arrival of
super-fresh fruit, vegetables and fish is treated as a special event,
with streamers and signs proclaiming 'Shun!'

To me, enhancing natural flavour means not smothering food
in heavy, creamy sauces, or salt, mayonnaise or ketchup, but using
gentle seasonings and light dressings that bring out the food's
original natural flavour.

The seasonings most commonly used in traditional Japanese
cooking are dashi cooking stock, sake, soy sauce, miso, mirin (a
sweet rice cooking wine), rice vinegar, sugar and salt. A Japanese

cook uses combinations of these seasonings in different numbers and quantities to achieve a desired flavour, taste and aroma.

My mother Chizuko's mantra, as she sprinkles sake or soy sauce into a saucepan on a stove, is *maroyaka,* meaning well rounded and mild. All the seasonings should be well blended and subtle, without any one taste screaming too loudly. Seasonings don't overpower the natural flavours of ingredients, no matter what you may be cooking: fish, vegetables or meat. When in doubt, use less seasoning.

The final point in the Japanese cooking philosophy, according to historian Ishige:

> *'What a cook must avoid is too much cooking.*
> *Japanese haute cuisine is based on the paradoxical cooking philosophy that the ideal way of cooking is not to cook.'*

When the ingredients are truly fresh and loaded with amazing tastes and textures from nature, you don't need to do much to them. Last week, I bought some ripe heirloom tomatoes at the height of their season from a stand at the Union Square Farmers' Market. Wow! The first bite filled me with such intoxicating flavours that I decided I should eat them plain. Even top-quality extra-virgin olive oil and balsamic vinegar would have been an insult to them. They were so hearty and meaty, they tasted like the earth and the sun.

Taken together, these insights explain why Japanese food can be so healthy and delicious. You can apply the ideas to any cuisine, not just Japanese food, and you can keep it in mind whether you prepare food at home, order at a restaurant, or buy takeaway or supermarket food.

Of course, you've got to cook meat and lots of other foods, and you can't always eat produce fresh from the fields, but I think if you favour fresh, natural foods gently prepared, you can't go wrong.

For decades, one of the top cooking oils used in Japan has been rapeseed oil, which is considered to be among the healthiest cooking oils because of its abundance of heart-healthy 'good fats' over 'bad fats'. Outside Europe, its counterpart is called 'canola oil'. In Japanese-style cooking, rapeseed oil is favoured over the almost-equally healthy olive oil because of its lighter taste.

> *A hand moves and the fire's whirling takes different shapes. All things change when we do.*
>
> – Kobo-Daishi
> Ninth-century Buddhist abbot

Another healthy Japan-style cooking method is simmering fish or sliced vegetables in broth, dashi or sake, often using a special wooden drop-lid called an *otoshibuta*, which helps broth distribute evenly and thoroughly among the ingredients, helps the ingredients maintain their shape and stay intact while they simmer, and requires less simmering time and cooking broth than using a normal lid.

Another distinct category of Japanese cuisine is vinegared dishes – often used for vegetables, sea vegetables and seafoods. Unlike their Western counterparts, traditional Japanese vinaigrettes do not include oil, thereby reducing calorie intake (see the recipe on page 170). The rice vinegar in Japanese vinaigrettes is mild, with only 4 per cent acidity compared to 6–8 per cent for wine or cider vinegar, and it's often diluted with dashi, making it milder, while adding subtle layers of flavour. The next time you think of making a salad, try the radish salad recipe on page 184. You can certainly substitute other veggies to make your own salad variations.

Japan Diet cooking spotlight: steaming

The technique of steaming, which originated in China, is a quintessential Japanese cooking method. It is such a gentle and healthy technique that it is recommended – along with boiling, poaching and microwaving – as a better alternative to frying or roasting food by both the Food Standards Agency and Heart UK. Steaming is a fantastic cooking method in my opinion for at least four reasons:

- It is a no-fat, no-oil method
- It retains the nutrients in food
- It liberates the natural flavours of food
- It can be super-convenient.

There are many different steamers to choose from – everything from little Chinese bamboo steamers, to high-tech electronic versions. Lately I've been using a fantastic, two-level stackable stainless steel steamer, which goes right on top of my stove, and I love it because I can steam lots of vegetables in no time.

I clean and slice the veggies, boil water in the steamer, drop in the veggies and they're ready in as little as five or 10 minutes. For vegetables such as spinach, kale and string beans, I immediately dip them in cold water to keep their bright green colours. I steam batches one after another, such as corn on the cob, followed by leafy greens and broccoli, and before I know it I have cooked more than enough vegetables for several meals. I often steam vegetables, squeeze out the excess water and toss them in a fragrant sesame seed dressing (see the recipe on page 172).

I think vegetables emerge from the steamer extra-delicious, and some vegetables, such as tomatoes get even sweeter. One trick is to slightly undercook them so that they are still crisp yet tender and their colours are bright. Sweet potatoes come out so sweet and hearty that I don't need to put anything else on them, such as salt or butter. Steaming fish keeps its flesh moist and tasty.

Eight Top Tips for Steaming Food

1. Consider investing in a simple, sturdy stainless steel steamer pot, with one or two vertically stacked steamer baskets, for your stove-top.
2. Clean and trim the veggies prior to steaming and cut into bite-size pieces.
3. Bring several centimetres of water to a rolling boil, turn the heat down to medium or medium-high and place chopped food in the steamer basket above the water. Allow some spaces among the vegetable pieces for steam to circulate. Make sure

the food is not sitting in water. During steaming, keep the cover on. Read the instructions for your steamer carefully.

4. For a rich flavour, add some fresh herbs to the steaming water, or place the food in a bed of seasonings and/or broth in a heat-resistant plate in the steamer.

5. Many veggies, when chopped into pieces, will steam at medium heat in roughly 5 to 7 minutes or less. Peas can take as little as 2 minutes, while a whole potato can take 15 to 20 minutes and a whole beetroot can take up to 35 minutes.

6. You can check for 'doneness' by pushing a fork or chopstick into the vegetable. It will be done when the fork pushes in easily, with little 'resistance'. Another guideline: when a vegetable releases its fragrance, it's close to being done.

7. Fish will steam in 4 to 12 minutes, depending on the type.

8. Be careful not to scald yourself when you uncover the steamer pot, as it can be really hot. Wear oven gloves, avert your face and lift the lid away from you.

DAY 18

LIGHTEN UP YOUR BEVERAGES

He grew up in a land of sugary drinks and deep-fried catfish.

As a child, he was stuffed full of food.

His family stuffed him with fried chicken, corn bread and mashed potatoes.

They stuffed him full of peach pie and home-made ice cream.

He got so fat that he was the only child at an Easter egg hunt to come up empty-handed, as he was too chubby to outrun any of the other kids. At the age of 15, he weighed 95 kg (15 stone). In college, the centrepiece of his first date with his wife to be was a super-sweet, caffeinated, carbonated beverage full of empty calories – Coca Cola.

His name was Bill Clinton.

When he prepared to enter the White House, Clinton was lurching at the gates of obesity, reaching a high of 102 kg (16 stone), despite regular jogging. The problem was that the jogging often ended up on the chow line at McDonald's, where he compulsively scoffed burgers, salted French fries and egg muffins. On the campaign trail, he was known to eat up to seven meals in one day.

In the Oval Office, when his wife was away, he ordered stacks of pizzas for himself and his staff from the local pizza place. For breakfast one day, he reportedly wolfed down eggs, venison sausage, pork sausage, 'scrapple' (fried pork scraps), bacon and ham, and had a lunch aboard Air Force One of brownies and turkey sandwiches. For dinner, he dived into some 'garbage pizza' (jalapeño peppers, olives, mushrooms, sausage – you get the picture) and topped it off with cheesecake and a cheese cannoli chaser. In between, he somehow managed to squeeze into a frozen yoghurt shop, where he asked, 'Can I have vanilla and strawberry, and some strawberry topping? Got any bananas? Put that in there, too.'

By the time he reached the age of just 58, former president Clinton's arteries were so severely clogged that his doctors reported over 90 per cent blockage, putting him in danger of a massive heart attack and in need of immediate surgery. Clinton's lifetime of poor diet habits, on top of what may have been a genetic predisposition for health risks, nearly killed him. It took a quadruple bypass operation, a 12-person surgical team and a heart-lung machine to repair the damage, rebuild his arteries and save his life.

But the former self-described 'fat band boy' Bill Clinton would soon exact a measure of revenge upon the demons of obesity. He declared war against the childhood obesity epidemic and in 2006 he persuaded the titans of Coca-Cola, Pepsi and Cadbury Schweppes to voluntarily ban selling sugar-sweetened fizzy drinks in all American primary schools, covering some 35 million children. 'This one policy can add years and years and years to the lives of a very large number of young people,' Clinton said.

In the UK, the campaign against sweetened fizzy drinks is becoming a mega-trend, and for very good reason. High intake of sugar-sweetened soft drinks probably increases our risk of weight gain and obesity, says the World Health Organization (WHO). The damage to children is particularly severe. Commenting on a WHO study of the links between chronic TV viewing and the rampage of childhood obesity, Dr David Haslam of the National Obesity Forum noted the 'disordered lifestyle' that many children are falling victim to. 'They sit in front of the telly with sweets, crisps and fizzy pop,' said Dr Haslam, 'and it's going to kill them.'

Japanese people consume lots of fizzy drinks, too. But remember, one of the most striking positive lessons of the Japanese diet is that, overall, the daily calorie supply per person of sugar in Japan is over 30 per cent less than in the UK.

Did you know that, according to the FSA:

- Adults and children in the UK eat too much sugar, and more of it comes from fizzy drinks than any other type of food or drink.
- Nearly 50 per cent of people in the UK consume fizzy drinks every day.
- Children who have lots of sugary drinks are more likely to put on weight and be overweight.
- Sugared fizzy drinks, squashes and 'juice drinks' contain lots of sugar – which means they contain a lot of calories – and very few nutrients. We should try to keep these to a minimum. The added sugar they contain can also damage teeth. Fizzy drinks fill us up, so we have less appetite for healthier foods.
- Food and drinks containing added sugars contain calories but few other nutrients, so we should try to eat these foods only occasionally. Cutting down on sugary drinks, such as cola and sweetened fruit beverages is a good way to reduce the amount of sugar you have.

Thanks to Jamie Oliver's school meals campaign and government crackdowns, UK schools have banned sugary fizzy drinks, along with crisps and chocolate, in their vending machines and tuck shops. The market for fizzy drinks has hit a wall, as consumers search for healthier choices.

> *Tea tempers the spirit and harmonises the mind, dispels lassitude and relieves fatigue; awakens thought and prevents drowsiness . . . its liquor is like the sweetest dew of heaven.*
>
> – Lu Yu, The Classic of Tea

Japan Diet spotlight: hot green tea and cold barley tea

One of the fastest-growing beverages in the UK is green tea. Its sales jumped over 300 per cent between 2000 and 2005, while sales of standard black tea dropped by 5 per cent over the same period.

In Japan, green tea has been a favourite all-day drink for many centuries, due to its clean, gentle, natural taste. It has less caffeine than coffee and is relaxing and soulful, like black tea. It comes from the same plant, too, only green tea is unfermented and therefore closer to the original *Camellia sinensis* leaves.

And unlike coffee and black tea, sugar and milk are almost never added to green tea, making it a low-calorie option, unless it is used to make sweets or desserts such as green tea custard pudding, green tea ice cream and green tea-flavoured biscuits.

The antioxidants in green tea have attracted a great deal of expert attention, and various health benefits have been claimed, including protection for the cardiovascular system and prevention of some kinds of cancer.

In 2005 and 2006, the US Food and Drug Administration rejected 'qualified health claims' that green tea reduced risk factors for cardiovascular disease and some forms of cancer, saying there wasn't enough evidence.

But in June 2006, a group of Yale University School of Medicine researchers published a paper in the *Journal of the American College of Surgeons* that said, 'The evidence is strong that green tea consumption is a useful dietary habit to lower the risk [of] and treat a number of chronic diseases,' and that 'the consumption of six to ten cups of tea per day might constitute an aid to increased health, longevity and quality of life'. And in September 2006, a questionnaire-based 11-year study of over 40,000 Japanese adults published in the *Journal of the American Medical Association* reported that those who drank lots of green tea – five or more cups a day – had less cardiovascular disease and lived longer than those who drank less than a cup a day. Definitive? Not necessarily, since the heavy green tea drinkers may have had other healthy habits. Interesting? Absolutely.

The research on green tea may be a mixed bag, but the taste can be fantastic. Try some Japanese green tea:

- Try a cup of hot green tea at the end of a meal, with or without dessert. It gives you the sense of a perfect finish. Or have a cup of hot green tea as an afternoon pick-me-up.
- Drink your green tea straight: no sugar, no milk. Don't be fooled by commercial gimmicks based on the green tea health craze. Stay away from sweetened and/or artificially flavoured green tea drinks, cold or hot. Look for all natural, unsweetened tea whenever you reach for a cup or bottle.
- Experiment and find your favourites: just like black teas, the higher the quality, the more superior your experience, and the better the aroma, flavour, texture and aftertaste. Try different labels and choose your favourites. Good green teas have mild, sweet, fresh tones. If a green tea is too bitter for you, it probably means that it's inferior or it's been steeped too long. If you just don't like the flavour of Sencha green tea, try Genmaicha, roasted brown rice and green tea, or Hojicha, a roasted green tea that has a more earthy flavour. Don't forget that green tea contains caffeine, though less than coffee.
- Try Mugicha, cold barley tea: Mugicha (pronounced 'moo-gee-cha') is roasted barley tea and is caffeine- and sugar-free. It is a refreshing, delicious cold drink with a naturally nutty-sweet flavour. When I was growing up in Japan, Mugicha was the *de facto* everyday, all-day cold beverage for the summer.

At a Japanese market or Japanese online store, you can buy a bag of Mugicha roasted barley tea bags. All you have to do is to drop a bag into a jug of water and let it steep in your refrigerator overnight – you will see the colour change to mild brown.

Try drinking Mugicha as an everyday cold beverage, instead of fizzy drinks. You can dedicate one jug for Mugicha (see the recipe below) and keep it in the fridge at all times. In between or during meals, whenever you're thirsty, have a glass. Here are some more beverage tips, from the Food Standards Agency:

Seven Top Tips on Healthy
Beverage Consumption

1. Drink 6 to 8 glasses (1.2 litres) of water, or other fluids, every day to avoid dehydration.

2. Drink plenty of water – the best choice for quenching your thirst between meals. It is totally calorie free and contains no sugars that damage teeth. Drink water or soda water, and zest it up with a wedge of lemon or lime.

3. Instead of sugary fizzy drinks and 'juice' drinks, go for cold water or unsweetened fruit juice (remember to dilute these for children). If you like fizzy drinks then try diluting fruit juice with sparkling water.

4. If you don't like the taste of plain water, try sparkling water, or add a slice of lemon or lime. You could also add some squash or fruit juice for flavour.

5. Remember that while 100 per cent fruit juices may have health benefits, they can also have a lot of calories. Check the labels to make sure there's no added sugar and watch out for 'juice drinks', which can be loaded with sugar and contain as little as 5 per cent fruit juice.

6. Sports drinks can be useful if you're doing endurance sports and need an energy boost. But often they're very high in calories. Unless you're taking part in an endurance sport, drinking water is probably the best way to re-hydrate.

7. For a healthy choice, choose semi-skimmed or skimmed milk. This is an important source of calcium, which helps to keep our bones strong. The calcium in dairy foods is easy for the body to absorb.

BREWING JAPANESE TEAS

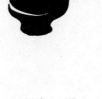

SERVES FOUR

SENCHA

4 teaspoons of loose tea leaves
450 ml (16 fl oz) of hot but not boiling water (about 80°C/175°F or
    bring the water to the boil and let it sit for 5 minutes before
    pouring)
Steeping Time: 1 to 1½ minutes

GYOKURO

7 teaspoons of loose tea leaves
450 ml (16 fl oz) of hot but not boiling water (about 60°C/140°F or
    bring the water to the boil and let it sit for 20 minutes before
    pouring)
Steeping Time: 2½ minutes

HOJICHA, GENMAICHA, OR GENMAIMACHA

3 teaspoons of loose tea leaves
450 ml (16 fl oz) of boiling water
Steeping Time: 30 seconds

Place the green tea leaves in a teapot. Pour the hot water (at the
temperature appropriate to the type you are serving) and let the
leaves steep for the time specified above. Since different varieties of

tea require amounts, water temperatures and steeping times that may vary slightly from my directions, please follow the directions on the package if they differ from mine. Lay out 4 teacups. Fill each cup one-eighth full, then make the round of the 4 cups again, filling them another eighth of the way. Repeat until you have used the very last drop of the brewed green tea. The point of doing this is to ensure that you are serving the same strength of tea to all your guests. The teacups should be filled half or two-thirds of the way to the rims. Do not leave any liquid in the teapot because the tea becomes bitter when it cools. You can reuse the same leaves for a second serving. Simply repeat steps 2 and 3 when you are ready to serve the next round of tea.

Cold Mugicha (Barley Tea)

Pop one Mugicha tea bag in a litre of cold water and let the mixture steep overnight in the   refrigerator. The next morning your Mugicha will be ready. (Each Mugicha brand may require a different amount of water and steeping time. Please read the directions on the package. Keep refrigerated.)

DAY 19

THE JAPAN DIET SHOPPING GUIDE

The Japan Diet is a series of choices. It is a gentle 'makeover' of your shopping decisions and your eating attitude.

To make the choices easy, one of the essential tricks is to surround yourself only with those foods that are good for you, so you can't go wrong whatever you reach for.

Here is a supermarket shopping guide to help steer you towards healthy choices, featuring some – but by no means all – of the items to choose more of, as well as items to choose less of. It is based both on the Japanese diet and on the advice of leading nutritional authorities.

Remember that a 'healthy, balanced diet', according to the FSA, includes meals based on starchy foods, such as bread, rice, pasta and potatoes – these types of foods should make up about a third of the food you eat; lots of fruit and vegetables, also making up about a third of your diet – aim for at least five portions of a variety of fruit and veg each day; plus some meat, fish, eggs or pulses (beans, lentils and peas).

And be 'nutrition-aware'. Learn to read food labels for nutrition facts and ingredients so you can keep a mental note of calories, fat, salt and sugar. Remember that nutritional information is given per serving and per 100 g. The ingredients are listed in order of quantity.

JAPAN DIET SUPERMARKET SHOPPING GUIDE

Choose More

Food items
- All fruits and vegetables

- Oily fish

- Other seafood
- Wholegrain breads, cereals and pasta
- Brown rice
- Unsalted nuts and seeds
- Rapeseed oil (non-hydrogenated)
- Olive oil, sunflower oil (non-hydrogenated)
- Lower-fat milk, yoghurt and cheese
- Lean cuts of meat and poultry
- Tofu (plain), edamame soya beans
- No- or low-salt vegetable stock
- No-salt flavourings such as lemon, herbs and spices
- Cold water as a beverage
- Bottled unsweetened green teas

Comments
- Choose many, from a wide variety of types and colours – they are low in calories and nutrient-rich
- Source of 'good' unsaturated fat, tinned versions are okay too, but look for lower-sodium choices
- Source of various nutrients
- Starchy foods, these contain fibre and various nutrients
- Good wholegrain source
- Source of 'good' unsaturated fat
- Source of 'good' monounsaturated fat
- Source of 'good' monounsaturated fat

- Less saturated fat

- Trim off any visible fat and remove skin
- Versatile protein alternatives to fatty meat, in moderation
- Healthy choice for cooking
- No sodium, add great aromas and flavours
- No-cost option: from your tap
- Refreshing, healthier option to fizzy drinks (may contain caffeine)

Choose Less

Food items
- Fatty meat, meat pies, sausages, streaky bacon, meat with visible white fat
- Hard cheese, such as Cheddar
- Butter and lard
- Pastry, doughnuts, cakes and biscuits

Comments
- High in saturated fat

- High in saturated fat
- High in saturated fat
- High in saturated fat, added sugar, may contain trans fats

• Cream, soured cream and crème fraîche	• High in saturated fat
• Coconut oil, coconut cream or palm oil	• High in saturated fat
• Foods with hydrogenated vegetable oil	• May contain trans fats
• Whole milk and dairy ice cream	• High in saturated fat
• Fizzy drinks, other sweetened drinks	• Often calorie dense/nutrient poor
• Creamy salad dressings and dips	• High in saturated fat
• Crisps, salted snacks	• High in salt, calorie dense/nutrient poor
• Ready meals and takeaway	• If they are high in salt, high in saturated fat, and if they contain few vegetables
• Fast food, especially fried	• High in saturated fat, calorie dense/ nutrient poor, may have trans fats, may be high in salt

Immerse yourself in a farmers' market

The farmers' market, in my opinion, is one of the most brilliant inventions of modern history. In 1997, the UK had only one farmers' market. Today there are more than 500 around the country, selling locally produced, super-fresh fruit and veg, organic produce, fish, lobster and crab, herbs, bread, juice, eggs, honey, preserves, wines, cider, beef, lamb, pork, poultry, preserves, cut flowers and plants.

You can actually talk to the farmer who grew your food! If you haven't sampled the pleasures of a farmers' market lately, I urge you to pay one a visit. It can be a fantastic experience. Visit each stall. Notice the seasonal vegetables and fruits and inhale the earthy aromas. Talk to the farmers; ask them for recommendations and tips.

On Saturday mornings in New York City, I visit the big, bustling Union Square Market, which is a brisk 2 km (1¼ miles) walk from our apartment. I like to get there in the morning, just after the lorries have been unloaded, when the seasonal produce is neatly piled, and plants and flowers are spread out, radiating intoxicating aromas and dazzling colours.

I love how the farmers' market reflects each season. Colours change dramatically, unlike the supermarket, which looks the same no matter which day of the year it is.

In winter months, the market is splashed with the earthen colours of root vegetables. Hot apple cider simmers in a big aluminium pot at the edge of the apple display. It's one of my favourite pick-me-up drinks on a cold morning. It is naturally sweet-sour, hot and punchy. I sip it slowly from the opening of the plastic top, inhaling its aroma. The cider warms and perks me up slowly, as I walk on to check out the next farmer's offerings.

In the springtime, the bright warm colours of flowers fill the grounds and I buy bunches of cut roses. Baby herbs fresh from the nurseries fill the tents and beg me to take them home. I grab the usual suspects: thyme, rosemary, basil, sage and oregano. In the summer, the market is even greener and more bustling. The strong sun sharpens the rich red colours of strawberries, cherries and tomatoes.

I love how most of the time veggies at a farmers' market have not been trimmed and you get to see them in their entirety. For vegetables such as carrots, beetroots and radishes, I like to eat the leaves, not just the roots.

A farmers' market is a perfect place to find your food, and you'll find information on where you can find one in your area in the resources section at the end of this book.

Pay a visit to a Japanese market

If you live in or near London, you've got some great choices for stores that sell speciality Japanese foods and other goods, such as The Japan Centre in Piccadilly, The Japanese Kitchen in Putney and the Rice Wine Shop and Arigato Japanese Supermarket, both on Brewer Street.

This week, why not step inside and have a look? Walk around the shop, explore the shelves and pick up a few simple 'starter' items such as:

- Short- or medium-grain rice, or sushi rice
- Dry soba buckwheat noodles (look for low-sodium, 80 to 100 per cent buckwheat)

- Mirin
- Sake
- Sesame oil
- Brown rice vinegar
- Lower-sodium soy sauce
- Red or white miso paste (look for lower-sodium versions)
- Instant dashi Japanese cooking stock
- Dashi ingredients (kombu, sea vegetable, and bonito, fish flakes) for making dashi from scratch
- White sesame seeds (whole and ground)
- Shredded nori sea vegetables, to sprinkle into soup or over rice
- Green teas (loose leaves and teabags)
- Mugicha, barley tea packets
- Shichimi, seven-flavour Japanese spice mixture

If there isn't a Japanese market within easy reach, you can surf some of the Japanese grocery websites in the resources section at the end of this book.

Time-saving short-cuts

I wish I had time to cook like a master chef all the time, but I don't. I buy fresh veggies and wash, trim, slice and cook them – but I also buy washed and ready-to-use vegetables, too. When I have time, I make dashi, the home-made traditional Japanese cooking stock, from scratch, but I also use instant dashi. In the office, I use more convenient green tea bags instead of the loose leaves that I have at home.

I don't have the time or skill to clean fish, so I always ask the fishmonger to clean it for me. Sometimes, just to save some time, I ask the fishmonger to de-vein and shell prawns while I shop in a different section of the market.

Here are some more short-cut ideas and products I usually try to have on hand, to save time or avoid a tedious task, and I'm sure you can find more:

- 90-second microwaveable plain brown rice pouches.
- No- or low-sodium vegetable stock in liquid form (I don't use cubes because they can be salty).

- No- or low-sodium fish stock in liquid form.
- Instant Japanese dashi cooking stock from a Japanese market or online store in granules, liquid or pouch forms. Look for no-monosodium glutamate (MSG) versions, if you prefer.
- Tinned Alaska salmon in water. I've always got some in my cupboard.
- Tinned sardines in water.
- Frozen, shelled edamame beans, a perfect snack or addition to many dishes.
- Frozen, steam-in-the-bag mixed vegetables.
- Tinned no-salt whole tomatoes.
- Marinara sauce in a jar.
- Pre-washed, ready-to-serve fresh baby spinach in an air-tight bag.
- Pre-washed, ready-to-serve fresh salad mix in an air-tight bag.
- Peeled, seeded, sliced, packaged fresh fruits, such as mangoes, papayas, watermelons and pineapples.
- Boned, skinned chicken.
- Boned, skinned, cleaned fish.
- Shelled, de-veined prawns/shrimps.
- Cooked plain prawns/shrimps.
- Bottled unsweetened green teas.
- Green tea bags.
- Clean and trim fresh vegetables, as soon as you get home, and store them in vegetable storage bags, which keep them fresh for longer, and label with name and date of purchase.
- Cook in bulk and refrigerate: for example, dashi, sauces, toasted sesame seeds, boiled/steamed vegetables.
- Cook in bulk and freeze: divide into single-serving portions, wrap and freeze, for example, rice, blanched (briefly boiled) vegetables.
- Online shopping – many Japanese staples are available online from Japanese grocery websites and, as you know, many regular supermarkets are offering online shopping now, too.

DAY 20

JUMPSTART WITH BREAKFAST

Did you skip breakfast today and go to work on an empty stomach?

Did you think that maybe that way you'd wind up eating a little less today?

I used to skip breakfast, too, out of sheer laziness, I'm afraid. But eating regular healthy breakfasts, it turns out, is a great way to help control your weight.

When I grew up in Japan, there was no way I could get away with skipping breakfast.

My mum cooked breakfast every morning. If I dashed out of the apartment without eating or drinking anything, my mum would literally chase me down the pavement in her apron, waving a piece of toasted bread in the air and exclaiming, 'Nao-chan! Have a bite, at least one bite! It's not good to go with an empty stomach!'

Years later, after I moved to New York, I got in the habit of skipping breakfast. It seemed like a hassle, and it felt like a better use of my time to race to the office, grabbing a cup of coffee on the way. Sometimes I wolfed down a muffin, or a bagel. Most of the time, though, I would nibble on my breakfast snack and, once absorbed in the day's work, forgot all about it, while the muffin or bagel sat there sadly on the corner of my desk going dry.

Then one day I awoke in Ballinalacken Castle in the little coastal town of Doolin, on Ireland's west coast, where I was attending a friend's wedding. I ordered a hearty traditional Irish breakfast, minus the bacon and sausages: poached eggs, halved and grilled tomatoes, toasted multi-grain bread, orange juice and coffee.

I gazed through the window; it was a crisp autumn morning and the sun was chasing away the mist over the Aran Islands and the Cliffs of Moher in the distance.

In that moment, I rediscovered the joys of breakfast. That meal changed my life. It was years ago, and I've had breakfast on most days ever since.

These days, I often have either a quick bowl of wholegrain oatmeal with some fruit, or my favourite morning meal: a bowl of vegetable and miso soup, a breakfast inspired by what my grandmother Tsune used to serve us when we visited her at her home in the Japanese countryside.

The ingredients change from day to day and usually include a bunch of grab-out-of-the-refrigerator ingredients stirred into a bowl of boiled water:

- Several bite-size cubes of firm plain white tofu.
- Some brown rice.
- 2–3 cherry tomatoes.
- A bite-size piece of sardine or salmon from a tin, or an egg.
- Generous amounts of whatever veggies are left over from the night before.
- Two teaspoons of miso paste, two flavours mixed: red miso and yellow miso.
- A sprinkling of shredded nori sea vegetables.

This is my simplified version of a traditional Japanese breakfast, where most of these items are served in separate bowls and dishes.

You may be thinking, 'is this woman completely loopy?' She has vegetable-soya-and-fish soup *for breakfast*? It might sound like a very weird idea.

But if you stop and think about it, it's not so off-the-wall. At some time you've probably had fish for breakfast, in the form of kippers, and may have enjoyed at least four veggies in the morning – beans, tomatoes, mushrooms and potatoes, for example. My Japanese breakfast is really just an expanded version of that.

The warmth, aromas and flavours of the soup wake me up slowly and gently, one spoonful at a time. By the time I slurp the last spoonful, I am wide awake, alert and energised. I am full, but just perfectly. I really like the feeling of how the soup fills me up, but doesn't weigh me down. And I am productive all morning. I also notice that now that I have three meals and one or two pieces of fruit a day, my lunches and dinners are often smaller than before, and I am comfortably full and totally satisfied throughout the day. You should give it a try!

In the UK, as many as 33 per cent of people are missing breakfast and it's happening in Japan, too. Some people think it's a way of reducing your daily calories, when in fact the opposite may be true. 'Research shows that eating breakfast can actually help people control their weight,' reports the FSA. 'This is probably because when we don't have breakfast we're more likely to get hungry before lunch and snack on foods that are high in fat and sugar, such as biscuits, doughnuts or pastries.'

The US National Institutes of Health agreed, declaring, 'Studies show that people who skip breakfast and eat fewer times during the day tend to be heavier than people who eat a healthy breakfast and eat four or five times a day.'

Beyond weight control, according to the British Dietetic Association, other breakfast benefits include improved health, mental performance and concentration, and a better mood.

The overall message is, it's not okay to skip breakfast. Nutritionally speaking, it is a pretty bad idea.

If you want to lose weight, eat a healthy breakfast!

Four Secrets to Long-Term Weight Loss from People Who've Actually Done it

The National Weight Control Registry (NWCR) is a database of over 4,500 adults who have successfully lost an average of over 27 kg (4 stone 4 lb) and kept the weight off for an average of over five years. The following behaviour was common to successful weight-loss maintainers:

1. Eating a low-fat, high-carbohydrate diet.
2. Regular self-monitoring of body weight and food intake.
3. High levels of physical activity.
4. Eating breakfast on a regular basis.

The Registry is supervised by Dr James Hill, of the University of Colorado, and Dr Rena Wing, of Brown University. They and their colleagues wrote in the journal *Obesity Research* in 2002 that according to self-reported questionnaires of members of the Registry, 'Eating breakfast is a characteristic common to successful weight loss maintainers and may be a factor in their success'.

They found it 'striking' that only 5 per cent of the successful dieters reported never eating breakfast, and speculated that 'eating breakfast may reduce the hunger seen later in the day that may in turn lead to overeating'.

Naomi's Quick Healthy Breakfast Options:

- Japan-inspired: bowl of low-sodium soup with added veggies.
- Japan-inspired: small bowl of short-grain rice (sprinkled with sea vegetables such as shredded nori if you like), a portion of veggies and a small piece of grilled fish.
- Japan-inspired: small bowl of short-grain rice, grilled tomatoes and a small piece of fish.
- A salmon sandwich (no mayonnaise) or sardines on wholegrain toast.
- Wholegrain cereal with sliced banana and a glass of fruit juice, or soya-based beverage.
- Multi-grain toast with sliced banana (see recipe page 214).
- Bowl of mixed fruit with low-fat unsweetened yoghurt.
- Bowl of low-fat muesli, wholewheat cereal or oatmeal with skimmed milk and fruit (for example, sliced banana, dried fruit, berries, half a grapefruit).

Your Japan Diet Small Shift

Skipping meals doesn't work. Eating a regular healthy breakfast can help me lose weight and power me into a bright new day.

DAY 21

INTEGRATE YOUR EXERCISE

Did you know that moderate exercise can be just as effective as intense exercise?

The old cliché 'No pain – no gain' is history. There's no need to torture yourself any more to get fit and fabulous. All you have to do is take long brisk walks in the fresh air.

It isn't often that you'll hear a doctor say, 'I was wrong,' but I know of one who did:

'I regret preaching the doctrine of aerobics as I did for so many years,' said Dr Harvey Simon, a Harvard Medical School associate professor, who in 1987 wrote a book called *The Athlete Within.* That book encouraged people to take up three to six hours of intense exercise per week.

But in 2006 Dr Simon revised his opinion, in a new book, *The No-Sweat Exercise Plan,* which makes a strong case for the benefits of lower-intensity exercise as well, such as walking, gardening, cleaning the house, taking the stairs and walking the dog at the end of the day, or dashing out for a lunchtime walk instead of staying in the cafeteria. 'You don't have to push yourself to get major health benefits,' he argued.

According to Dr Simon Till, chair of the British Association of Sports Medicine, 'Five or 10 minutes of moderate-intensity exercise done several times a day will give you excellent fitness benefits.' For example, Dr Till reported in the *Daily Telegraph of* 11 March 2006, only three 10-minute spurts of medium-intensity exercise per day, like walking briskly to the paper shop so your heart rate is raised sufficiently, 'will improve your cardiovascular and respiratory health, lower your risk of diabetes and other diseases and improve your longevity, irrespective of whether you lose weight'.

When I lived and worked in Japan I seemed to walk everywhere. And I believe it contributed to my healthy weight loss.

In the morning I walked 15 minutes to the tube station, then up and down a flight of stairs to the train. It's rare to get a seat during peak hours, so I would be standing, either listening to some music on my personal stereo, or reading a paperback book, for an average of 30 minutes.

I'd get off at the main Tokyo Station downtown and take another 10- to 15-minute walk out of the station to my office and repeat the process. For lunch, my colleagues and I walked a couple of blocks to a nearby local restaurant. When we went out in the evening, we would take a tube train and then walk several blocks to a bar or restaurant. Between stairways and the labyrinthine walkways in and out of the trains, I was getting nearly an hour's workout every day. And I was usually moving pretty fast, so that I wouldn't be late for work or late at my mother's dinner table.

I didn't belong to a gym and I wasn't playing sports regularly, but I had an 'incidental' work-out automatically plugged into my daily life, whether I liked it or not. On weekends, I escaped the densely populated central Tokyo area and rambled around the tranquil pathways of Kamakura, a historic city dotted with shrines, temples and gardens.

This lifestyle was a huge change from my chubby period as a student in the USA. When the dorm was closed during holidays and I stayed with a local family, I sometimes hardly moved. When we went out, we'd step straight into the garage, which was a part of the house, and get into the car. When we returned, the driver pushed a button and the garage door opened automatically and we just rolled into the garage. Out of the car and into the house, in less than 10 steps! Now that I live in New York City, I'm walking as much as I did in Tokyo.

The idea of 'integrative exercise', or the everyday physical activity we build into our daily lives, is attracting lots of excitement from researchers and they are seeing many benefits, not just in aerobic activity, but in moderate exercise.

It's part of a trend among diet experts that sees physical activity as a fully integrated part of a healthy diet. 'Now there's a big push in the nutrition field to consider both food and activity to be nutrition,' said Dr Ann Yelmokas McDermott, research scientist at Tufts University. 'It's the energy balance equation: "energy in", in the form of foods and calories, and "energy out", in the form of structured exercise, daily living and physical activity.'

'People don't fail in losing weight, they fail in keeping it off,' said Jim Hill, professor of medicine at the University of Colorado. 'We see it over and over, the key to long-term success is the ability to ramp up your physical activity.'

In Japan, surprisingly few adults belong to fitness clubs and people are becoming more sedentary than they used to be, yet the nation has the longest healthy life expectancy in the world. One reason could be that Japanese people still enjoy more integrative exercise in their daily routine than people in the West, with relatively more walking and bicycling and less time behind the wheel of a car.

A study published in the 1 November 2005 issue of the *Journal of the American College of Cardiology* lends support to the idea that Japanese health advantages are not all genetic. The report, based on questionnaires of 73,000 adults in Japan aged 40 to 79, found that even in an Asian nation where people are believed to have higher levels of job-related physical activity than in Europe or North America, those who walk more or engage in regular sports activity tend to have lower levels of ischaemic stroke and coronary heart disease than Japanese people who are less active.

We live in an 'obesinogenic' society that seems geared to removing physical activity from our lives. 'The everyday lives of most people are almost as if they were in a coma,' said registered dietitian Robyn Flipse. 'They are in their cars, at their desks, in front of computers, in front of TV screens. They push a button to microwave their food, to wash the dishes, to do the laundry, to turn on the TV.'

Dr John Buckley, spokesman for the British Association of Sport and Exercise Sciences, reported that, 'The activity levels of people in the 1950s was equivalent to walking three to five miles a day because they did not have the equipment and devices we have today.' What's changed, said Buckley, 'is the lack of short bouts of lower-intensity activity in our daily lives'.

It is no good squeezing all this extra activity into your day if you eat more than you need. But cut down on the calories you consume, accumulate more activity throughout the day and you are guaranteed to lose weight.

– Louise Sutton
Senior Lecturer, Sports Nutrition
Leeds Metropolitan University

The health benefits of regular physical activity are remarkably rich and varied, affecting how much we weigh, how we feel and how long we live. According to the World Health Organization and the National Health Service, regular physical activity:

- Helps control weight and appetite, and lowers the risk of becoming obese by 50 per cent compared with people with sedentary lifestyles.
- Promotes psychological well-being, reduces stress, anxiety and depression.
- Reduces the risk of dying prematurely.
- Reduces the risk of dying from heart disease or stroke, which are responsible for one-third of all deaths.
- Reduces the risk of developing heart disease or colon cancer by up to 50 per cent.
- Reduces the risk of developing Type 2 diabetes by 50 per cent.
- Helps to prevent/reduce hypertension, which affects one-fifth of the world's adult population.

- Helps to prevent/reduce osteoporosis, reducing the risk of hip fracture by up to 50 per cent in women.
- Improves strength, flexibility and balance; helps build and maintain healthy bones, muscles and joints, and helps people with chronic, disabling conditions improve their stamina.
- Can help in the management of painful conditions, such as back pain or knee pain.

One of the easiest and most effective forms of exercise, when done regularly, is what we've been doing all our lives, without any special equipment or training – namely walking. According to Dr JoAnn Manson, chief of Preventive Medicine at Brigham and Women's Hospital, 'Walking is an accessible, inexpensive and virtually injury-resistant form of physical activity that confers enormous health benefits.'

To see how effective walking and other exercises can be, take a look at these examples, which show the approximate number of calories burned by a 70 kg (11 stone) person doing the named activity at moderate intensity or speed:

Physical Activity	Time taken (minutes)	Energy used (calories)
Walking	60	250
Cycling (at 10 mph)	30	200
Swimming	20	190
Gardening	30	180
Ballroom dancing	30	155
Aerobics	20	150
Sweeping the floor	30	90
Weight lifting	20	75

Tips for boosting and integrating your exercise lifestyle

Here are some ideas for working more physical activity into your life. They include my tips, plus suggestions from the Department of Health, the US Institutes of Health and other experts. Always consult your doctor before starting an exercise programme.

- The combination of a reduced-calorie diet and increased physical activity is recommended since it produces weight loss that may also result in decreases in abdominal fat and increases in cardio-respiratory fitness.
- All adults should set a long-term goal to accumulate at least 30 minutes or more of moderate-intensity physical activity on most, and preferably all, days of the week. This regimen can be adapted to other forms of physical activity, but walking is particularly attractive because of its safety and accessibility. The important thing is to find something you enjoy and do it safely.
- Getting started: you can start out by walking 30 minutes for three days a week and can build to 45 minutes of more intense walking, at least five days a week. With this regimen, you can burn 100 to 200 calories more per day.
- Try to make physical activity a way of life – for good. Make it a regular and enjoyable part of your day.
- Take a 10-minute walk after breakfast, lunch and dinner to reach the goal of 30 minutes per day.
- Take short stretch breaks throughout the day and go for a walk.
- Park your car at the far end of the car park as a regular habit.
- Walk briskly at the shopping centre or mall, especially in bad weather.
- Walk (or even jog) some of your shorter journeys.
- Run around and play with your children for 30 minutes a day.
- Think of ways of becoming more active that you will enjoy, such as dancing, bowling or gardening.
- Mind and body exercise alternatives to traditional exercise provide variety and fun. They may also help reduce stress, increase muscular strength and flexibility and increase energy levels. Examples of these exercises include yoga, Pilates and tai chi.
- On holiday, include activities that require more than just sitting by a pool or on the beach: go rambling in the

countryside, go to a historic place that offers lots to see on foot (not just a museum), take a guided walking tour and/or spend time at a working farm.

- Participate in volunteer projects. Clean a park, beach, footpaths, streams; plant flowers and shrubs in a park.
- Physical activity may include structured activities such as walking, running, basketball, or other sports. It may also include daily activities such as household chores, gardening, or walking the dog.
- Set short-term and long-term goals and celebrate every success.

Track your progress

- Keep a physical activity diary and write down when you worked out, what activity you did, how long you did the activity for, and how you felt during and after your workout. You can make a note of opening times, and special sessions, at the swimming pool or planned events, such as an organised walk.
- Use a pedometer. This is a gadget that fits onto your belt and counts the number of steps you take. Many people have found a pedometer keeps them motivated to walk more each day and helps them set new goals. You can buy a simple, inexpensive pedometer from your local chemist or supermarket.
- Aim to increase the number of steps by, say, 1,000 every few days. Gradually build it up so that you are doing more and more steps each week. Adults can work towards a goal of 10,000 steps a day.
- At the end of each month that you stay on your exercise programme, reward yourself with something new – clothes, music, art, or a book – something that will indulge you and help keep you committed. But don't use food as a reward.
- Get a friend or family member to join you and motivate each other to keep it up.

Dr Denise Simons-Morton is Director of the Clinical Applications and Prevention Program of the Division of Epidemiology and Clinical Applications at the US National Heart, Lung and Blood Institute. She explained: We know that physical activity is a key lifestyle component that helps people control their body weight. I think the availability of an excellent public-transportation system is key to promoting physical activity during one's daily life.

In the well-populated areas of Japan, there are terrific public-transportation systems. People in the physical activity field have a saying that goes something like this: 'A public-transportation trip is a walking trip', because one must walk to and from (and between) public transportation sites.

Eating slowly in a relaxing atmosphere, having meals full of seafood, vegetables, soya and rice or noodles, along with copious amounts of walking during the day – these are lifestyle components that can be adopted widely for healthful effects.

Exercise Log

For the week of: ....

Day	Type of Exercise (weights, aerobic, other)	Duration	Intensity (minimal, challenging, strenuous)	Goal Accomplished (yes or no)	Notes
Monday					
Tuesday					
Wednesday					
Thursday					
Friday					
Saturday					
Sunday					

DAY 22

THE PORTABLE JAPAN DIET

When you're away from home, it can seem really hard to eat healthily, especially when you're travelling.

But it's easier than you may think.

You can take The Japan Diet with you wherever you go.

The key step is to remember the foundations of the healthy eating patterns we've explored together:

- Shop, order and eat mindfully.
- Load up on a wide variety of fruit and vegetables.
- Favour fish, oily fish, lean meat and poultry, starchy foods and wholegrains, and enjoy healthy, moderate, 'human-size' portions.
- Favour foods that are closer to nature, prepared and served in healthy ways.
- Lighten up your beverages.
- Avoid saturated fat, sugar and salt – no more than 6 g of salt a day.

You can apply these lessons to any food you enjoy – British, Indian, Italian, Japanese, French, regional dishes or any other cuisine.

Last year, we were invited to Australia and New Zealand by our publisher and the SunRice company to promote our book *Japanese Women Don't Get Old or Fat*. In Auckland, we found a New World supermarket near our hotel with a Japanese grocery section, and a few blocks away was a full Japanese grocery store called Japan Mart. Combined with the rich variety of local restaurants, seafood, meat and produce, it was all we needed to eat really healthily.

We took two weeks off to explore New Zealand's spectacular South Island, so we rented a cottage in Queenstown, which is about as far away from my home kitchen as I could get.

I felt like I was at the furthest end of the earth, but I was delighted to find a gourmet grocery store, called Mediterranean Market, that had just about everything we needed to turn a Kiwi kitchen instantly into a Tokyo-style kitchen. There were fresh organic vegetables in a temperature-controlled room, tofu, a basic selection of Japanese ingredients and seasonings, such as miso paste and sesame oil, and pouches of microwaveable medium-grain brown rice.

The healthy lessons of the Japan Diet are easy to bring along with you, whenever you're eating out at a restaurant, packing some snacks in your bag or going on a trip.

Here are some portable healthy eating tips, including some of my ideas and some suggestions from leading nutritional authorities.

Eating away from home, Japan Diet-style

No matter where you are going, do some advance research on the Internet to find local grocers, supermarkets, takeaways and restaurants that cater to your Japan Diet style.

Once you have a list of potential restaurant selections that you think will make a delicious healthy meal, ask the following questions by email or phone (you can add or subtract questions from the list):

The Japan Diet restaurant diner's Bill of Rights

- Do you have full nutritional information for all the dishes you serve? Very few restaurants do this yet, but I think it's time we started requesting it.
- Exactly how is the dish prepared? Is there a 'heart-healthy' option?
- What dishes are low in saturated fat and salt and free of trans fats?
- Can you avoid butter and use less oil when cooking my dish?
- Do you have wholegrain bread or cereals?
- Can you prepare my food with the least amount of sodium, added salt, MSG, or salt-containing ingredients?

Be mindful

When you are selecting a place to order a meal, remember to be mindful throughout the process:

- Select a store/restaurant that will accommodate your Japan Diet style of eating.
- Look for quality, not quantity.
- Stay away from 'all you can eat' deals, including sushi.
- Avoid buffets; order *à la carte* from a menu.
- Order a moderate portion for each meal.
- Think of vegetables as the main course and reverse the proportions of red meat and vegetables; instead of a huge chunk of steak and a small side dish of vegetables, choose red meat in smaller quantities and make vegetables the main part of the meal.
- Choose fish, especially the kinds that are rich in omega-3s, such as salmon, mackerel and sardines.
- Choose dishes that are steamed, simmered, poached, roasted, baked or grilled without oil or butter, rather than deep-fried, and choose garden-fresh or raw fruit and vegetables where possible.
- Choose dishes that are flavoured with fresh herbs and enjoy the natural flavour of ingredients and subtle seasonings.
- When ordering dishes that are cooked with oil, check that they are prepared with a small amount of rapeseed, olive or non-hydrogenated vegetable oils.
- Ask for sauces and dressings as a side order – not on the meal already – and use in moderation.
- Avoid excess animal fats, such as the fat on meat and the skin on chicken. Think of cheeses and red meat as occasional treats, instead of daily staples, and as flavouring/garnish, instead of main portions.
- Choose wholegrain foods.
- Say no to sugary fizzy drinks with your meal and ask for water with a slice of lemon and teas without sugar or milk.
- Make sweets and high-calorie puddings a more occasional treat and ask for small portions. Ask for fruits, nuts and seeds for snacks and desserts instead.

- Enjoy the meal: admire the presentation and tableware, savour every bite.
- Take time: put your utensils down after a few bites.
- Share your meal, order a half-portion, or order a starter as a main meal.
- Take half or more of your meal home. You can even ask for your half-meal to be boxed up before you begin eating so you won't feel forced to eat more than you need.
- Stop eating when you begin to feel full. Listen to your body.
- Focus on enjoying the setting and your friends or family for the rest of the meal.

Bend the rules

Rather than ordering a big main meat course at a restaurant, order several appetisers as your whole meal; or ask for a starter-sized portion of the main course, plus a salad and two starters. Whether you're eating with one person or a group of people, you can try sharing many of the dishes. It is a great way to:

- Have many more varieties of food instead of a large amount of one.
- Have a moderate portion for a meal.
- Try out new dishes.

Here are some examples of how you may structure a meal for two people:

Conventional

Each person orders one starter, one main course, one side dish and a dessert.

Japan-Diet style

- *Option 1*: Order three or more starters and a side dish (depending upon portions) between the two of you.
- *Option 2*: Order one or two starters, a side dish (depending upon portions) and one main dish between the two of you.
- *Option 3*: Order one or two main dishes (depending upon portions) and share both between the two of you.

Be aware of portion sizes

I've noticed that in the West even Japanese restaurants serve larger portions than their counterparts in Japan. Just because you're at a Japanese restaurant it does not mean that the balance of food you order is automatically healthy – big portions of foods that are deep fried or drenched in teriyaki or soy sauce are no more nutritious choices than bad Western food would be. Look at the volumes of food being served to other diners and adjust your order accordingly.

On-the-go snacks

Keep a bottle of water or unsweetened tea in your bag and pack in a small food storage bag or container with some of the following:

- Veggie sticks: carrot, peppers (green, red, orange, yellow), cucumber, celery, courgettes, radishes, broccoli and/or cauliflower florets.
- Steamed veggies: sweet potatoes, corn, broccoli and/or cauliflower florets.
- Seasonal fresh fruit: bananas, clementines, mandarins, peaches, plums, apples, sliced melon and/or pineapple.
- Handful of dried fruit.
- A few unsalted peanuts, almonds or walnuts. Nuts are a good source of fibre, vitamins and minerals and protein. Enjoy unsalted nuts in small portions, e.g. 15 g (½ oz) of nuts contains about 270 calories.
- Low-fat unsweetened yoghurt.
- A slice of wholegrain bread with a thin slice of low-fat mozzarella cheese, a wholegrain sandwich without mayonnaise, or a slice of wholegrain toast with banana and a little honey.
- Handful of unsalted rice crackers or rice cakes.
- Cottage cheese and plain cream crackers.

When travelling

- For a trip that starts early in the morning, take a bottle of water and one or two items from the above on-the-go snack list for breakfast/snacks rather than an overpriced airport/railway station fast food selection (or lack thereof!), or a minuscule airline breakfast.
- For room service, order the 'heart-healthy' options if available.

For the office

- Take one or two servings of fruit to work every morning. Get them fresh from a fruit trader's stall and put them near your workspace. When you feel like chewing something, reach out for a piece of the fruit that's right in front of you.
- Take along any one or two items from the above on-the-go snacks list.
- Keep a bottle of water or unsweetened tea by your side at all times. Stock your drawer with top-quality tea bags.

A JAPAN DIET-INSPIRED 7-DAY SAMPLE HEALTHY EATING PLAN

For when you have no time to cook, and barely time to shop!

You and I live in the BlackBerry world. It is a world of frantic schedules, demanding bosses and ultra-hectic family life. There's no way we're going to find the time to shop and cook from scratch every day.

I rarely switched on an oven until a few years ago, when I discovered the pleasures of cooking recipes from my mother's little Tokyo kitchen. Before that, I relied mainly on microwave and takeaway meals, restaurants, or a few simple cooker-top standbys such as spaghetti. But now I cook using fresh ingredients, as much as I can, often several times a week, because I find it soothing, therapeutic and relaxing. The whole process of shopping for fresh, beautiful ingredients at a market is reassuring and empowering, since I know what goes into my meal.

Washing, chopping, stirring and tossing the ingredients works as a stress-reliever for me and prolongs the joys of the simple act of eating. I enjoy the colours, aromas and noises during the course of cooking. I hum along to the sounds of chopping vegetables. I listen to the sizzle of a juicy fish fillet. I bury my face in a bouquet of herbs and inhale. I love the way the aromas of simmering dashi Japanese cooking stock fills the house. I watch the soba buckwheat noodles dance as soon as I release them into a large pan of boiling water.

I encourage you to try to cook at least once a month or better yet, once a week. You can experiment with some of the Japan-style recipes and sample meals I have put together for you at the end of this book.

But what do you do tonight, on the way home from work, if you're tired, you're late, you're hungry and all you want to do is relax with your family or crash out on your own with a good meal?

I have great news for you.

To enjoy the lessons of The Japan Diet, you don't always have to cook from scratch.

You don't have to learn how to cook Japanese food if you don't want to.

In fact, when you don't have time to, you don't really have to cook much at all.

All you have to do is stop at your local supermarket and make some good choices from the healthy ready meals, and supplement them with high-convenience 'grab and go' items.

It is getting easier and easier to eat healthily – and one reason is that supermarket ready meals are getting more nutritious.

We asked food expert Dr Frankie Phillips to explore the UK supermarkets for us. She is a registered dietitian and spokesperson for the British Dietetic Association. We asked her to visit Sainsbury's, Tesco and Waitrose stores to find out what healthy meal choices are available and how these supermarkets manage nutritional labelling.

Here's some of what she told us about ready meals:

> Look into the healthier options of those ready meals. Look for the lower-fat, lower-salt options and supplement them with a portion of vegetables on the side.
>
> Most supermarkets now offer a range of 'healthier' foods. Choose these but, crucially, supplement them with a portion of vegetables or a side salad as a really useful way of getting some of your five portions of fruit and vegetables. It fills out the meal, too.
>
> Some of these ready meals can actually be quite small portions, so by having the extra portion of vegetables, it does give you a feeling of really having eaten a proper meal.

It takes next to no time to prepare. Get a handful of frozen vegetables from the freezer and put them in a pan of boiling water for 2 minutes. While you're waiting for the ready meal to heat up in the microwave, you could easily be preparing yourself a side portion of vegetables to go along with it.

We also asked Dr Phillips to construct a sample meal plan for a week of super-convenient healthy eating, inspired by the best lessons of the Japanese diet and balanced nutrition.

Here is her report on supermarket healthy ready meals, followed by the sample healthy eating plan. Why don't you discuss this plan with your doctor or dietitian? It could be a convenient way to start easing into a lifetime of healthy eating!

A Dietitian's Analysis of Supermarket Healthy Ready Meals

This report was compiled by Dr Frankie Phillips, Registered Dietitian. The views expressed are based upon the professional considerations of the author as an independent UK registered dietitian.

All information is based on data collected from Waitrose, Sainsbury's and Tesco stores using information and products available in-store and online and the responses provided by their customer helplines.

Requests for further details were sent directly to the named nutritionists at each of the stores included in the report. Despite direct requests and further prompting, none provided any further information. In terms of policies, therefore, the information is based on that available to the author online, in-store and via the customer helpline.

From a dietitian's perspective, is there a wide selection of healthy ready meals available? What are the healthy ready meals called? What is their definition of 'healthy'? Do they have nutritional 'traffic lights' on the packet? In all three of the supermarkets studied, there is a reasonably good selection of healthy ready meals, suiting a variety of tastes. There is a range of cuisine, including Indian, Italian, British, Japanese, Chinese and vegetarian. Additionally, there is a good range of vegetables and salads that are ready to eat/cook/microwave and these can be used to supplement a healthy ready meal.

Waitrose – 'Perfectly Balanced'

The Waitrose healthy range of products is termed 'Perfectly Balanced' and has a distinctive livery on the packaging throughout the range. The range is said to be developed to strict nutritional criteria to help contribute to a healthy daily diet. There are more than 170 products in the range, including ready meals, sandwiches, cooking sauces and desserts. 'Perfectly Balanced' products are 3 per cent fat or less (therefore the whole range can be called 'low fat'), restricted in sodium (salt) content, free from artificial colours and sweeteners, and restricted in the use of all other additives.

The Waitrose 'Perfectly Balanced' range also claims to make no compromise on taste, portion size or ingredient quality. The number of calories per serving is highlighted on the front of pack, and there is a nutrition information panel on the back.

Waitrose are committed to using the FSA-recommended 'traffic light' labelling scheme, which was launched in March 2006. The separate traffic lights are shown on the front of the pack for fat, saturates, salt and sugars, alongside the amounts of each nutrient per portion. Calorie content per portion is also shown and the nutrition information is listed in table format on the back of the pack along with the guideline daily amounts (GDAs). At the time of the report, the traffic light labels are used on own-brand sandwiches and are being rolled out to ready meals, including those in the 'Perfectly Balanced' range, and pizzas.

Sainsbury's – 'Be Good To Yourself'

The Sainsbury's healthy range is called 'Be Good To Yourself'. Healthier choices can be identified by the presence of an apple logo on a pack. This is Sainsbury's symbol of health. The packaging is also identified by a consistent colour scheme.

The products in the 'Be Good To Yourself' range fall into one of three categories: 'Less than 3 per cent fat'; 'Healthier option', which has fewer calories, salt and saturated fat than the standard product lines; and 'Plus' products, which are fortified with added ingredients, such as probiotics ('friendly bacteria' for a healthy digestive system) and omega-3 fatty acids. The label states which of these criteria are met by the product.

In terms of nutritional labelling, Sainsbury's have declared that they are committed to helping customers follow a healthier lifestyle. As a part of this commitment, the 'Wheel of Health' traffic light labelling system was introduced in January 2005 and is in accordance with the recommendations of the Food Standards Agency. The 'Wheel of Health' shows the number of calories, and the amount of fat, saturates, salt and total sugars in one portion. The colour corresponds to high (red), medium (amber) or low (green) levels per 100 g (3½ oz) of the product.

Further details are usually available on the back of pack, showing Guideline Daily Amounts of the nutrients included in the 'Wheel of Health'. It also provides values for nutrients such as fibre and some vitamins and minerals. The 'Wheel of Health' is being rolled out to all own-brand products (not including staples such as butter and sugar, and children's products) and is already used widely on ready meals. The 'Wheel of Health' also appears on the 'Be Good To Yourself' range – all products in the range show green and amber, except for products that contain 'healthier' fats (that is from nuts and seeds) or high sugar levels from fruit.

Tesco – 'Healthy Living'

The Tesco healthy ready meals are termed 'Healthy Living'. The Tesco concept of the 'Healthy Living' brand states that 'You don't have to make dramatic changes to enjoy a healthier balanced diet'. The range includes more than 500 products including low-fat cuts of meat, convenience foods, and healthier versions of spreads, drinks and snacks.

These products contain either less than 3 per cent fat (along with a flash stating 'less than 3% fat') or half the fat of a Tesco standard product; contain either 10 per cent less sodium than a Tesco standard product or are already low in sodium; contain no more added sugar than a Tesco standard product. 'Healthy Living' ranges are available in most of the departments.

Tesco have made it clear that they do not support the policy of multiple 'traffic light' labels as recommended by the FSA and have launched a front-of-pack nutritional signpost system based on Guideline Daily Amounts (GDA) for an adult. The signposts show the amount (in grams) of salt, fat, saturates, sugar and the calories in a serving of each product, and also show the percentage of the GDA that a serving of the product contains. Tesco states that they are committed to putting clear front-of-pack labelling on all own-brand products by January 2007. The system is available on a range of products including the 'Healthy Living' brand.

Are there any glaring errors or improvements you see in overall presentation of the ready meals?
With respect to the healthy varieties of the ready meals reviewed for this report, the portion sizes would be appropriate for an average adult female, but would need to be supplemented (for example, with an additional slice of bread or side serving of potatoes) in many cases to provide sufficient for an adult male who did not need to lose weight. Many of the ready meals contained only small amounts of vegetables. Some did not include vegetables at all. However, some of the products included serving suggestions, such as also buying a side portion of salad or vegetables.

In all cases, labels had to be read carefully as the healthy option was not always 'low fat' or 'low salt'. The use of 'healthy' branding implies that they are a healthier option in all respects, but they are not necessarily always, for example, low in fat. This may be rather confusing to the consumer who is trying to select a low-fat and low-salt diet.

With regards to salt content, this is probably the most challenging area in attempting to meet current recommendations of no more than 6 g salt per day. Although manufacturers and retailers are recognised as making moves to reduce the salt content of their products, there is still some way to go. The 'healthy eating' ranges of all the supermarket brands studied include reduced sodium as one of the criteria, but these products often still fall into the medium- or high-salt content classifications outlined by the FSA.

In addition, own-brand supermarket ready meals may have a very different labelling system from that of outside brands, such as McCain, Birds Eye or Heinz. This makes it more difficult to compare at a glance own-brand with premium-branded ready meals.

Are the ready meals sold in microwave-ready containers? Do many of them take just a few minutes to heat up?
Ready meals are sold in microwave-ready containers, and cooking instructions are given, based on cooking the product in its container (for example, pierce the film cover before microwave heating). The microwave-ready meals do take only a few minutes to heat up and instructions for cooking from frozen or chilled, using microwave ovens of different wattage, are provided. A small range (such as Sainsbury's 'Just Cook') are not suitable for microwave cooking, and some ranges are only suitable for oven cooking (for example, pizzas).

Is there a pre-made sushi section, how extensive is it and what are your impressions of it? Is the sodium content listed on the packet?
All supermarkets have a pre-made sushi selection, which is presented alongside sandwiches. The selection is quite small in many cases and a 'healthy eating' range is not available. Vegetarian and fish options are available and most packs of sushi have a small portion of soy sauce to add. The sushi has nutrition labels with sodium and salt content listed, although this may not be on the front of pack.

Are there nutritional 'traffic lights' on all other food items in the store?
No, the extent of use of nutrition 'traffic lights' is currently limited to a range of own-brand products in those stores where the system

is being used. Food items displaying the colour coded 'traffic lights' system include ready meals, sandwiches and breakfast cereals, as well as products that are labelled as the 'healthy eating' range. Currently, Sainsbury's has the most extensive use of the traffic light system, using its 'Wheel of Health' colour coded logo – this is used on a wide range of own-brand products.

Manufacturers including Kellogg's, Kraft, Nestlé and Pepsico all use the GDA system of labelling and are unlikely to adopt the FSA system of 'traffic light' labelling. These products are in stores alongside own-brand labelled products.

In addition, many products sold loose (such as deli and bakery items) do not necessarily carry any nutrition information labels. It was recently announced that two other UK retailers, ASDA and Co-Op, will be introducing the 'traffic light' labelling scheme on own-brand products.

Is the fresh produce section extensive?
In most UK supermarkets, the fruit and vegetables section is located at the front of the food department and generally covers approximately 10 per cent of the total floor space. The selection is usually good, with a wide range of produce from basics to 'exotic' fruit produce.

Are there many pre-packed fresh salads and veggie platters?
Each supermarket has a good range of pre-packed fresh salads, both unwashed and ready to eat. Some are prepared as 'ready meal' salads (for example, tuna layered salad in a pot, or Healthy Living Caesar Salad). Prepared vegetables are widely available, but few are presented as crudités or vegetable platters.

Is there an Asian or Japanese food section?
All supermarkets studied had an Asian (Japanese, Chinese and Thai – South East Asian) food section, and an Asian section of ready meals, both chilled and frozen. The Asian foods section typically consists of rice, noodles, sauces, some canned vegetables and condiments. Tesco and Waitrose had a very small (one or two

shelves only) selection of Japanese foods within the Asian foods section, whereas Sainsbury's had a 'speciality products' section including a flip chart of products available from diverse regions of the world – Italy, Greece, Indonesia and Japan. A similar selection was available in all of these supermarkets.

Availability of some sample Japan-style staples

• Microwaveable plain brown rice	• Uncle Ben's microwaveable wholegrain rice is available in Tesco, Sainsbury's and Waitrose.
• Short-grain white rice in a bag	• Sushi rice is available in the Japanese foods section in Waitrose, Tesco and Sainsbury's.
• Refrigerated unsweetened Japanese tea	• Pokka Japanese Green Tea is available in Waitrose.
• Tofu – unflavoured, refrigerated	• Cauldron brand available in unflavoured packs refrigerated in Waitrose, Sainsbury's and Tesco.
• Lower-sodium soy sauce	• 25 per cent lower-sodium soy sauce is available in Tesco, Waitrose and Sainsbury's.

Sushi choices in UK retail outlets are usually limited to ready-made packs made using white rice and containing relatively high levels of sodium. A small number of takeaways – mainly located in London – can prepare sushi to order using a choice of fish and vegetables or tofu.

How difficult or easy is it today for a consumer to get healthy, nutritious food in the supermarket?
In the current climate where convenience rules many peoples' food preferences, owing to great pressures on time, it is becoming increasingly easy for a consumer to have a healthy diet, based on the choices that they can make at the supermarket. However, for

those trying to follow a low-salt diet, it is necessary to spend a little more time reading the labels, particularly where front of pack labelling is not available.

Overall, health does not need to be sacrificed in the quest for convenience, and supermarkets have a huge part to play in helping people to make the transition to healthier choices, whether this is done overtly, by making labels easier to understand, or covertly, through changing taste preferences by gradually reducing, for example, the salt content of regular bread.

Pricing policies that favour healthier choices (for example, buy a healthy ready meal and get a free bag of salad), improved labelling and providing a good range of quality basic produce ensures that supermarkets provide the essential components of a healthy, nutritious diet.

In terms of labelling, the development of a clear and consistent way of highlighting how much fat, sugar and salt there is in a food will make it much easier for people to put healthy eating advice into practice when shopping.

It is the role of the supermarket to ensure that the components of a healthy diet are available, and supermarkets are making moves to improve access to a healthy diet for all, but it is ultimately the responsibility of the consumer to select the products that will contribute to a healthy, nutritious diet.

A Dietitian's 7 Day Sample Healthy Eating Plan Based on Healthy Ready Meals and Supermarket 'Grab-and-Go' Items

This seven-day meal plan is based on a range of ready meals, takeaway and 'grab-and-go' foods that are readily available in Waitrose, Tesco and Sainsbury's stores, at the time of writing, plus sushi choices from these stores or a sushi takeaway.

The menus are based on the principles of a healthy diet, including white fish, oily fish, lots of vegetables and salads, lean meat and poultry, wholegrains, fruit, nuts and yoghurts for snacks and desserts, and low-sodium, low-sugar and low-saturated fat choices, where possible.

The menu plan is suitable for an adult male or female. Slightly larger portions of rice, noodles, potatoes, bread and breakfast cereals should be selected by males who do not want to lose weight.

Each day should include at least 1.5–2 litres (2½–3½ pints) of healthy drinks, such as water, unsweetened tea and green tea and an allowance of approximately 300 ml (½ pint) semi-skimmed (or skimmed) milk or an equivalent amount of calcium-fortified soya milk.

Snacks can be consumed at any time of the day.

Day	Breakfast	Lunch	Evening Meal	Snacks
Sunday	Porridge (cook in microwave) made with semi-skimmed milk with 1 tbsp of raisins 1 slice wholemeal toast with 1 heaped tsp no added sugar/salt peanut butter Small glass pure orange juice	Sainsbury's Be Good To Yourself Salmon in watercress sauce with a large portion of steamed broccoli and carrots, served with brown rice (e.g. ½ a 250 g pack of Uncle Ben's microwave wholegrain rice)	Waitrose Perfectly Balanced Lasagne Salad of baby leaves, grated carrot and beetroot, sesame seeds and lemon juice 2 kiwi fruit	Apple 3 dried apricots ½ packet Sainsbury's Almond Berry mix (almonds, cranberries, raisins)

Day	Breakfast	Lunch	Evening Meal	Snacks
Monday	Tesco Healthy Living muesli with mixed fresh berries and fat-free natural yoghurt Small glass pure apple juice	Sushi – made to order – brown rice (if available) with cucumber and fresh tuna or crayfish and avocado – no added salt or soy sauce (or Tesco medium sushi pack – no soy sauce added) Sainsbury's Be Good To Yourself Cucumber and Pomegranate side salad (with yoghurt dressing)	Sainsbury's Be Good to Yourself Thai Green Chicken Curry with jasmine rice served with steamed pak choi 1 pear	6 fresh lychees ½ Toasted wholegrain bagel topped with 1 tsp peanut butter and chopped banana

Day	Breakfast	Lunch	Evening Meal	Snacks
Tuesday	2 Shredded Wheat with sliced apple and semi-skimmed milk Small glass of Tesco Finest Mango, orange and banana smoothie	3 Waitrose Perfectly Balanced no-added-salt rice cakes each topped with 1 tbsp of Tesco Healthy Living cottage cheese and pineapple Tesco fresh superfruit salad	Sainsbury's vegetable kebabs served with microwave wholegrain rice (½ of a 250 g pack) (e.g. Uncle Bens) Tinned peaches in juice served with 1 pot Tesco Healthy Living fromage frais and 1 tbsp chopped mixed nuts	2 plums Handful of cherry tomatoes 3 walnuts

Day	Breakfast	Lunch	Evening Meal	Snacks
Wednesday	Porridge (cook in microwave) made with semi-skimmed milk with 1 tbsp of raisins 1 banana Small glass pure grapefruit juice	Waitrose Perfectly Balanced King Prawn Noodle Salad Small bunch black grapes	Waitrose Perfectly Balanced Vegetable Korma with Pilau Rice served with a cup (140g) of steamed broccoli, or string beans (e.g. Waitrose frozen or fresh vegetables) Baby leaf salad with grated beetroot and carrot Waitrose Perfectly Balanced fruit yoghurt	1 orange 1 slice wholemeal toast with 1 heaped tsp no added sugar or salt peanut butter 3 dried figs

Day	Breakfast	Lunch	Evening Meal	Snacks
Thursday	Tesco Healthy Living muesli with semi-skimmed milk 1 peach Small glass cranberry or pomegranate juice	Waitrose Perfectly Balanced Prawn and Poached Salmon Sandwich Sticks of fresh carrot and celery with 1 tbsp Tesco Healthy Living Hummus dip 2 plums	Waitrose Perfectly Balanced moussaka served with a side salad of mixed leaves 1 pot Tesco Healthy Living fromage frais with chopped banana	10 fresh cherries 3 dates ½ packet Sainsbury's Almond Berry mix (almonds, cranberries, raisins)

Day	Breakfast	Lunch	Evening Meal	Snacks
Friday	2 slices wholegrain toast with 1 small tin Waitrose Perfectly Balanced baked beans Small glass pure grapefruit juice	Sushi – made to order – brown rice (if available) with cucumber and fresh tuna or crayfish and avocado – no added salt or soy sauce (or Tesco medium sushi pack – no soy sauce added) 1 pear	Sainsbury's Be Good To Yourself Easy Steam Salmon Fillet with Tarragon served with a portion of ready prepared noodles e.g. Amoy and a large portion of spinach (fresh or frozen) Sainsbury's Be Good to Yourself fruit yoghurt	3 dried apricots 3 brazil nuts 2 passion fruit

Day	Breakfast	Lunch	Evening Meal	Snacks
Saturday	2 Shredded Wheat with semi-skimmed milk Small glass pure orange juice	Tesco chickpea dahl (ready to eat) 1 pot with selection of deli bar salads (mixed leaf, cucumber, carrot, beetroot, tomato) and yoghurt dressing	Waitrose Perfectly Balanced cod served with wholegrain rice (e.g. 125 g Uncle Ben's microwave rice) and steamed green prepared vegetables (e.g. mange tout, broccoli, green beans) Sliced melon	3 walnuts ½ a fresh diced mango 1 apple

Author's note: other supermarket food ranges that are being positioned as healthy choices include ASDA's 'Good for You', Marks & Spencer's 'Eat Well' and 'Healthily Balanced', Somerfield's 'Good Intentions', Morrisons' 'Eat Smart' and Co-op's 'Healthy Living'.

Food Standards Agency criteria for 'traffic light labelling'

Per 100 g criteria proposed:

	LOW	MEDIUM	HIGH
Fat	3 g or less	3.0–20 g	20 g or more
Saturates	1.5 g or less	1.5–5 g	5 g or more
Salt	0.3 g or less	0.3–1.5 g	1.5 g or more
Sugars	5 g or less	5–22.5 g	22.5 g or more

Per portion criteria proposed for foods eaten in quantities greater than 250 g:

	HIGH
Fat	21 g
Saturates	6 g
Salt	2.4 g
Sugars	27 g

Note: no criteria are given for calories to be included in the Traffic Lights Labelling Scheme.

DAY 30

THE DAYS OF MAGICAL EATING . . .
AND AN ETERNAL LOVE AFFAIR
WITH FOOD

When with the first month comes the spring,
Thus breaking sprays of plum-blossoms,
We'll taste pleasure to the full.
- POEM COMPOSED AT A MEDIEVAL JAPANESE BANQUET

When I was a girl, my grandmother Tsune took the overnight train
from her farm in the country to visit my family in Tokyo.

As I remember one of these visits now, it seems like a kind of
summit meeting of the Japanese home chefs.

My grandmother was an original 'Earth Mother', a full-time
farmer and mum with smiling, twinkling eyes whose skin was
tanned from endless hours in the fresh air. She cooked
delicious, simple, 'old-school' meals from ingredients fresh
from the family farm: eggs from the chickens in the garden,
vegetables from the hillside, rice from the fields and tangerines
from the groves.

My mother Chizuko is a city girl and also a master home cook,
who has blended many global influences into her repertoire.

I remember one evening when Tsune sat at our table and
watched Chizuko bring out a plate of spaghetti with tomato sauce,
something that was completely new to Tsune. She bowed to the
table and quietly announced, 'I am so grateful to receive this dish
that I have never tasted before in my life.'

Then she repeated an old Japanese saying, 'A new food prolongs one's life.'

She said this every time she tasted a new food during her visit. And she bowed again, murmuring, 'I am so grateful. So grateful.'

Through the magic of their home cooking, these two women inspire me today to have an eternal love affair with healthy food.

The gift of food is a gift of health and love that's contagious. My mum Chizuko has shown her love to her husband Shigeo, my little sister Miki, and me through all the meals she has prepared.

She often makes statements like, 'Health is one of the most important things in life. Without it, life is not worth living. Without it, you can't enjoy life. Eat delicious healthy foods, otherwise you won't be able to accomplish anything.'

She showered her love on my husband Billy through a symphony of home-cooked meals he'd never tasted before, and literally changed his life in the process, by converting him, without even trying, to a new lifetime of healthy flavoursome eating.

I would love to take you to Tsune's farm and Chizuko's kitchen, so you can taste and smell and feel the warmth and goodness of their versions of The Japan Diet.

I would love to take you on a tour of the Japanese mountain valleys and fields blanketed with fresh fruit and vegetables, the cities overflowing with gourmet food and the tiny home kitchens blossoming with the intoxicating flavours of home-cooked food.

Japan's food culture has been changing and, sadly, not all for the better. But the wisdom and the lessons remain, just below the surface and around a nearby corner. 'Many curious and beautiful things have vanished,' wrote Lafcadio Hearn over a hundred years ago, 'but old Japan survives in art, in faith, in customs and habits, in the hearts and homes of the people: it may be found everywhere by those who know how to look for it.'

The goodness of The Japan Diet and other healthy traditional diets lies all around us, in the choices we can make every day at our supermarkets, farmers' markets, restaurants and takeaway shops. It's right in our hands.

Tonight, let's celebrate our journey together by making a quick dinner inspired by The Japan Diet.

Naomi's Quick and Easy Japan-style 30 Minute Dinner Menu To Celebrate Your New Lifetime of Healthy Eating

SERVES 2

- Firm tofu with spring onions
- Simmered mixed vegetables
- Alaska salmon
- Brown rice
- Miso soup with baby spinach
- Fruits for dessert
- Green tea

FIRM TOFU WITH SPRING ONIONS

Time 2 minutes

125g (4 ½ oz) firm plain tofu

2 tbsp chopped spring onions, rinsed under water and drained

1. Drain and cut the tofu into bite-size cubes.
2. Arrange on an individual small plate, garnish with 1 tbsp chopped spring onions. Serve chilled, but not ice cold.
3. Let each diner drizzle over 2–3 drops of reduced-sodium soy sauce (optional).

SIMMERED MIXED VEGETABLES

Time 15 minutes

1 kg (2 lb) mixed colourful fresh vegetables such as onions, carrots, broccoli and sweet potatoes, or your choice of seasonal vegetables
700 ml (25 fl oz) lower-sodium vegetable stock, pre-made dashi, or instant dashi

1. Slice the veggies into bite-size pieces, setting the broccoli florets aside.
2. In a medium saucepan, simmer all the veggies except the broccoli florets in the vegetable stock on medium-high heat for 3 minutes, or until the broth simmers, covering the contents with a drop-lid (see page 232). Turn down the heat to medium and simmer for 10 minutes, or until the veggies are crisp yet tender and not mushy.
3. Add the broccoli florets and cover with the drop lid to coat the florets with the cooking broth. Simmer for another 1 minute, until the florets are bright green and crisp yet tender.
4. Arrange a moderate portion of the colourful veggie chunks in medium bowls and spoon over a small amount of broth.

ALASKA SALMON

Time 2 minutes

140 g (5 oz) tinned Alaska salmon in water
¼ lemon
1 tbsp chopped coriander leaves

1. Drain the water from the tin and arrange equal portions of the salmon on two microwaveable plates. Cover and microwave for 30 seconds.

2. Squeeze a little lemon juice over the salmon and garnish with chopped coriander leaves. Don't worry about the skin and little bones in Alaska salmon. They are completely edible and nutritious.

BROWN RICE
••••••••••••••••••

Time 90 seconds approx.

••••••••••••••

A pouch of 90-second microwaveable brown rice
••••••••••••••

While you are simmering the vegetables, microwave the brown rice and serve it in its own bowl, without any oil or butter.

MISO SOUP WITH BABY SPINACH
•••

Time 8 minutes

••••••••••••••

750 ml (1 ¼ pint) pre-made dashi (see page 168) or instant dashi (see page 169)

4 tsp lower-sodium miso paste (white or red, or both)

100 g (3 1/2 oz) baby spinach leaves

••••••••••••••

1. Cut the spinach leaves into 2-cm (¾-in) strips.

2. In a small saucepan, bring 750 ml (1¼ pint) dashi stock to boil and then reduce to medium heat. Dissolve the miso paste in

the broth. Add the spinach leaves, stir and turn off the heat. Serve immediately.

DESSERT

•••••••••••••

•••••••••••••

Seasonal fresh fruits of your choice
Green tea (unsweetened bottled cold tea, or hot steeped tea)

•••••••••••••

Presenting and enjoying the meal

Remember to leave some empty space around the food. Lay out the meal on the table as if it were a painting. If you've got some chopsticks around the house, great – but they're optional. A fork, knife and spoon are fine. Take a moment to admire the meal in front of you and take a moment to congratulate yourself on your achievement. Eat a little of this, a little of that, sip some soup and move slowly from dish to dish. Put your utensils down in between bites and sips.

Savour every bite. Take note of the beautiful colours, shapes and smells. Let the beauty of the food slowly take over the rest of you.

Relax, take your time and inhale the rich flavours. Indulge yourself with the fresh mature taste of the green tea, the cool subtle texture of the tofu, the perfectly cooked rice and the full-bodied soul-warming miso soup.

Help yourself to a second bowl of veggies or brown rice, if you like.

Finish off the meal with the seasonal fruit and a cup of freshly brewed tea.

You're now totally full and satisfied.

Mmmm! A dinner fit for a princess. That's a Zen Food Moment. Thank yourself for this beautiful moment.

In less than 30 minutes, you have created a healthy, delicious, classic home-cooked Japan-style dinner: a soup, three side dishes and a bowl of rice, plus some fruit and tea for dessert.

The meal you prepared is similar to the meals that Japanese people have been enjoying for hundreds of years.

Your Japan-style dinner is packed with flavour and it is on the cutting edge of the world's hottest dietary trends. It's loaded with nutritional buzzwords – it is low-GI and low calorie-density, it is nutrient-rich and full of antioxidants, phytonutrients, isoflavones, wholegrains, fibre, good carbohydrates and good fats.

In 1988, when I moved to the USA for the second time (this time New York) I consciously and unconsciously devised a way of eating that mirrored my roots in Japan, a way of eating that made me feel fantastic inside and out.

I did not have an exact formula and I wasn't trying to lose weight. I just wanted to eat delicious food and feel good.

I simply followed my intuition and craving, and somehow recreated the kinds of meals I would have had in Japan, out of Manhattan grocery stores, delis, cafés and restaurants. I figured it out as I went along. Food was not my main focus or concern. My work and life was.

I find Japanese-style eating to be really easy, even though I live in a highly Westernised city like New York, with tasty junk food everywhere. But I feel so good and energetic when I eat Japanese-style that the junk food doesn't stand much of a chance.

I have been eating mostly this way now for years. When I came to New York, I was 28 years old, weighed 47 kg (7 st 5 lb). Today, I am 46 and I weigh 49 kg (7 st 10 lb), which feels good and comfortable to me, and is a 'normal' body mass index, or BMI.

I am not skinny.

I don't want to be stick-thin or hollow-cheeked, I just want to feel fantastic and enjoy life.

Like anyone else, my weight fluctuates by a few kilos. When I am super busy, I lose a couple of kilos and I don't need to step on a scale to know it. I can feel it. My trousers are slightly baggy and I have extra room under my arms.

During the winter months, because of New York's severe freezing weather, when we are buried in snow, I don't get to walk so much and I crave comfort foods. Days are shorter, I stay in longer, then I gain a couple of kilos. I try to imagine that the little extra weight I feel around my body is the extra layer of clothing, but I know better.

When I feel that I'm putting on a few kilos, my internal scale gets switched on and starts blinking signs at me: 'I don't feel good – feed me with good food!' I listen and slightly adjust my eating and exercise behaviour to feel great again.

Through the experience of getting fat in America and losing the extra weight through the Japan-style diet with virtually no effort, I accidentally became a conscious, mindful eater.

As the poet Basho wrote, 'Learn all the rules, then forget them.' In other words, let the lessons of healthy eating become second nature to you. They are not a set of rules to make you feel stressed or anxious or guilty, but an everyday, natural attitude of living.

Forget about losing a few kilos, for now.

Just focus on how you feel – listen to your body.

I predict that when you start eating healthily, you will start feeling great. Your mind becomes clearer. You have more energy. You feel cleaner and lighter, and you'll want to keep doing it. It's a positive addiction. You will be leaner and healthier. You will feel, sound and look more fantastic.

Do it little by little. Take small steps, one at a time. It should be a gradual transformation. Be mindful, selective, demanding and finicky about the quality of foods and drinks you put in your mouth.

Enjoy your food with all your senses. Try new vegetables and fish and foods you've never had before. Try different combinations of veggies. Try new restaurants and order new dishes. Try new exercises and sports. Experiment with new techniques, tips and short-cuts.

Get into the rhythm of the Japan Diet attitude day in and day out; three or more meals a day. Fine-tune your techniques. Deconstruct. Improvise. Practise balance and moderation. Read up on the latest scientific discoveries on nutrition and health, and incorporate new insights into your diet.

If you stay with it, you will suddenly see the heavy clouds part and realise you have been steadily climbing and have come to a high mountain ridge. Turn around and see how far you have come. Look out and see the brand new landscape that spreads in front of your eyes.

Can you believe how magnificent the view is? You have created it.

There is no end to this journey. You will keep on going for more magnificent views. The Japan Diet is an art that you can strive to perfect without an end to come. In the meantime, it will propel you to a beautiful sphere in many aspects of your life that you can't even imagine today.

Share your love of healthy eating with your partner, children, family and friends. It is an eternal love. You have just begun the voyage.

Eat for your body to function beautifully. Eat to nourish your body, mind and soul. Eat to live well and eat to live a long, healthy life.

Don't do it just because it's healthy.

Do it because it feels fantastic!

SAMPLE JAPAN DIET MEALS BASED ON RECIPES

Here are some sample Japan-style meals you can construct from the Japanese recipes that follow. They are designed to achieve an overall good mix of both land and sea vegetables, rice/wholegrains, oily fish, soya, fruits and tea.

Each meal also employs varied cooking methods, tastes and textures to make it exciting.

You can add your own recipes that follow the Japan Diet principles to keep this eternal journey fresh and full of new discoveries on the way. These sample meals and recipes can serve as inspirations for you to come up with entirely new ideas of your own.

BREAKFAST 1
3-minute Breakfast: Miso Soup with Extra Firm Tofu &
    Spring Onions
Fluffy Japanese Rice (Brown, White or Haiga)
Green Tea or Mugicha

BREAKFAST 2
Cauliflower–Napa Cabbage 'East-Meets-West' Soup
Fluffy Japanese Rice (Brown, White or Haiga)
Green Tea or Mugicha

BREAKFAST 3
Miso Soup with Wakame Sea Vegetable &
 Spring Onions
Fluffy Japanese Rice (Brown, White or Haiga)
Green Tea or Mugicha

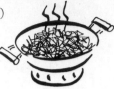

BREAKFAST 4
Scrambled Tofu with Salmon
Miso Soup with Wakame Sea Vegetable &
 Spring Onions
Fluffy Japanese Rice (Brown, White or Haiga)
Green Tea or Mugicha

BREAKFAST 5
Very Berries: Strawberries, Blueberries &
 Raspberries
Toasted Multi-grain Bread
Miso Soup with Extra Firm Tofu &
 Spring Onions
Green Tea or Mugicha

LUNCH 1
Seared Jumbo Prawns on a Bed of Mesclun Salad
Rice with Edamame Soya Beans
Miso Soup with Clams & Mitsuba
Green Tea or Mugicha

LUNCH 2
Grilled Portabello Mushroom Open Sandwich with
 Creamy Tofu Sauce
Sliced Seasonal Fruits
Green Tea or Mugicha

LUNCH 3
Chicken & Eggs (Parent & Child) over
 Fluffy Rice

Miso Soup with Wakame Sea Vegetable &
    Spring Onions
Green Tea or Mugicha

Lunch 4

Soba Buckwheat Noodles with Shiitake, Crimini
    Mushrooms & Garlic Sauce
Miso Soup with Extra Firm Tofu & Spring Onions
Cold Mugicha

Lunch 5

Beef, Sweet Potato & Onion Casserole – One Pot Dish
Kinpira Carrots with Hot Chilli Peppers
Fluffy Japanese Rice (Brown, White or Haiga)
Miso Soup with Extra Firm Tofu & Spring Onions
Green Tea or Mugicha

Dinner 1

Seafood Medley over Sushi Rice
Asparagus Salad with White Sesame Dressing
Miso Soup with Extra Firm Tofu & Spring Onions
Sliced Seasonal Fruits
Green Tea or Mugicha

Dinner 2

Grilled Salmon, Broccoli & Onions over Fluffy Rice
    (Brown, White or Haiga)
Steamed Veggies with Ginger Soy Sauce
Sautéed Beetroots
Miso Soup with Extra Firm Tofu &
    Spring Onions
Sliced Seasonal Fruits
Green Tea or Mugicha

Dinner 3

Vegetable Gyoza Dumplings

Edamame Mesclun Salad
Fluffy Japanese Rice (Brown, White or Haiga)
Miso Soup with Clams & Mitsuba
Sliced Seasonal Fruits
Green Tea or Mugicha

DINNER 4

Lightly Sautéed Five Colour Veggies & Tofu Chunks: Broccoli,
    Carrot, Onion, Yellow Courgette & Red Bell Pepper
Simmered Bass in Mild Teriyaki Sauce
Radish Salad
Miso Soup with Wakame Sea Vegetable &
    Spring Onions
Fluffy Japanese Rice (Brown, White or Haiga)
Sliced Seasonal Fruits
Green Tea or Mugicha

DINNER 5

Japanese Country Style Simmered Chicken, Broccoli & Carrot
Fluffy Japanese Rice (Brown, White or Haiga)
Miso Soup with Extra Firm Tofu & Spring Onions
Sliced Seasonal Fruits
Green Tea or Mugicha

SNACK 1

Sliced Fuji Apples with Cheeses
Gyokuro Tea

SNACK 2

Steamed Sweet Potatoes
Sencha Tea

SNACK 3

Hand to Mouth – Ready to Eat Fruits: Strawberries,
    Cherries, Plums, Grapes, Bananas
Hojicha Tea

SNACK 4
Very Berries: Strawberries, Blueberries & Raspberries
Genmaicha Tea

SNACK 5
Bananas on Toasted Multi-grain Bread
Cold Mugicha

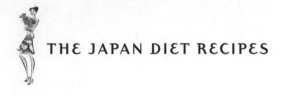

THE JAPAN DIET RECIPES

Here is a treasury of recipes for you to enjoy as you start to explore the delicious new thinking of the Japan Diet. In our previous book *Japanese Women Don't Get Old or Fat: Delicious Slimming and Anti-Ageing Secrets*, I introduced you to more than 30 traditional home-cooked recipes from my mother Chizuko's Tokyo kitchen.

If you have been to Japan, an authentic Japanese restaurant outside of Japan, or if you're familiar with traditional Japanese home-cooked meals, you'll know that the dishes I chose for that book, such as beef over rice, spinach with bonito flakes, kinpira, cold soba buckwheat noodles, are staples of a traditional Japanese menu.

They are quintessential Japanese, just like roast beef and Yorkshire pudding, roast potatoes, pork chop, shepherd's pie and beans on toast are for the British, and meatloaf and mashed potatoes with gravy, and burgers and fries are for Americans.

Every Japanese family has their own version of these recipes. Not only are they standard Japanese home-cooked dishes, they are also all-time favourites of mine that my mum cooked for me when I was growing up, and again when I went back to Tokyo after spending two years in the USA – and she still does.

They were the dishes that I wanted to be able to recreate for myself, my husband Billy and my American family and friends. I also made sure that the dishes were relatively easy to make, even if you know nothing about Japanese cooking, and that most people will enjoy eating. In case you haven't read our first book, here we reprise a couple of basic recipes from that book, such as dashi cooking stock, Japanese-style rice, and brewing green teas, as well as the Tokyo kitchen key ingredients, and add over 40 new recipes.

A note on conversions

Metric and imperial measurements are given in the following recipes. The two are not exact conversions, however, so please follow one or the other but do not mix the two in the same recipe.

COOKING STOCKS

JAPANESE VEGETARIAN (SHIITAKE MUSHROOM) COOKING STOCK

Makes 450 ml (¼ pint)

10 dried shiitake mushrooms, rinsed to remove any debris, especially from the stems
500 ml (18 fl oz) cold water

1. Place the shiitake mushrooms in a medium saucepan. Add the cold water to the saucepan, bring the mixture to the boil, immediately turn off the heat and let the mushrooms rest in the liquid for 15 minutes.
2. Pour the stock through a fine-mesh sieve lined with muslin. Drain the shiitake mushrooms, squeeze gently to remove excess water. Cut off and discard the stems. Leave to cool and store in a refrigerator for up to a few days.

Dehydrated mushroom caps (once pre-soaked) can be used in a variety of dishes, such as soups, sautéed vegetables, simmered vegetables and noodle sauce.

DASHI – JAPANESE FISH COOKING STOCK

FIRST DASHI

Makes 900 ml (1 ¹/₂ pint)

One 10 x 10-cm (4 x 4-in) sheet kombu (sea vegetables)
1 litre (1 ³/₄ pints) cold water
24 g (1 oz) large bonito flakes

1. Place the sheet of kombu in a medium saucepan. Do not wash or wipe off the whitish powder on the seaweed's surface, it abounds with natural minerals and flavour. Add the cold water to the saucepan and bring the mixture almost to the boil. Immediately remove the kombu (saving it for making second dashi) to avoid the liquid becoming bitter.
2. Add the bonito flakes and heat the liquid on high. When the stock returns to the boil, immediately turn off the heat and let the flakes rest in the liquid for 2 minutes. Pour the stock through a fine-mesh sieve lined with muslin. Avoid pressing on the flakes, to prevent the stock becoming cloudy and bitter. (Save the bonito flakes for second dashi.)
3. Leave to cool and store in the refrigerator for up to two days (it spoils quickly).

SECOND DASHI

Makes 900 ml (1 ¹/₂ pint)

1. Combine the 'used' kombu and bonito flakes from making the first dashi in a medium saucepan. Add 1 litre (1 ¾ pints) of cold water and bring the mixture to the boil. Reduce the heat to low and simmer for 10 minutes.
2. Pour the stock through a fine-mesh sieve lined with muslin, discarding the solids this time. Leave to cool and store in the refrigerator for up to two days.

Japan Diet Short-cut

As a quick alternative, you can use instant dashi Japanese cooking stock sold at a Japanese grocers. It comes in liquid, pouch or granulated forms. Please read the pack label to make sure that it is lower in sodium, and if you prefer, ask for a version that contains no MSG. Each form and brand differs in its preparation and use, so please read the directions on the packet.

You can use pre-made Western-style low-sodium vegetable stock/broth, or fish broth/stock instead, if you like. The flavours and textures of the dishes will be different from the ones cooked using Japanese cooking stock. Please make sure it is low-sodium since standard pre-packed products tend to be quite salty.

DRESSINGS, SAUCES &
MARINADES

SESAME OIL SALAD DRESSING

Makes 100 ml (3 fl oz)

40 ml (3 tbsp) rice vinegar
3 tbsp minced red onion
1 tsp sugar
15 ml (1 tbsp) toasted sesame oil
Pinch of salt and freshly ground black pepper

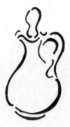

In a small bowl, whisk together the vinegar, red onion and brown sugar until the sugar is dissolved. Whisk in the sesame oil and season with a generous pinch of salt and several grinds of pepper.

TRADITIONAL JAPANESE VINAIGRETTE

Makes 100 ml (3 fl oz)

80 ml (6 tbsp) brown rice vinegar
4 tsp sugar
$^1/_2$ tsp sea salt
1 tsp low-sodium soy sauce

In a small bowl, mix the ingredients until the sugar is dissolved.

CREAMY TOFU SAUCE – YOU'LL NEVER GO BACK TO MAYO

Makes 180 g (6 oz)

150 g (5 ¹/₂ oz) firm tofu, water drained
2 tbsp Dijon mustard
Pinch of sea salt
Juice of ¹/₂ lemon (or 1 tbsp)

In a food processor bowl, blend all the ingredients until smooth. Transfer to a serving jar. Store the sauce in an airtight container in a fridge for up to two days.

TOASTED & GROUND WHITE SESAME SEEDS

Makes 40 g (1 ¹/₂ oz)

40 g (1 ¹/₂ oz) white sesame seeds

Pre-heat oven to 180°C/350°F/Gas 4, spread a single layer of sesame seeds on a baking sheet, cook for 1 minute (watch that they don't burn), then transfer the seeds to a suitable container, to avoid further cooking. Grind the toasted sesame seeds in a seed grinder, or mortar.

WHITE SESAME SEED DRESSING

Makes 200 ml (7 fl oz)

40 g (1½ oz) toasted ground white sesame seeds (see above)
80 ml (3 fl oz) dashi (see page 168)
80 ml (3 fl oz) low-sodium soy sauce
2 tbsp sugar

In a small bowl, blend the toasted, ground seeds, dashi, soy sauce
and sugar well.

RICE DISHES

RICE WITH EDAMAME SOYA BEANS
•••

Makes 1 kg (2 lb)
••••••••••••••••

370 g (13 oz) Japanese short-grain rice (white)
570 ml (20 fl oz) water for white rice
225 g (8 oz) frozen shelled edamame soya beans

••••••••••••••••

1. Wash the rice according to the instructions for fluffy rice (see page 97).
2. To cook the rice, transfer the washed grains to a medium saucepan. Add 570 ml (20 fl oz) cold water and leave the rice to soak for 20 minutes until plump.
3. Add the edamame soya beans over the rice. Do not mix the rice and the beans.
4. Cover the saucepan and bring the rice to the boil. Reduce the heat to low and gently simmer the rice for 15 minutes, or until all the liquid has evaporated. Turn off the heat and let the rice sit, covered, for 10 minutes.
5. When ready to serve, fluff the rice grains and edamame beans by gently turning them over with a wet wooden, or plastic, rice paddle.

SALMON CHAHAN (FRIED RICE)
•••

Serves 2
••••••••••••••••

3 tbsp rapeseed oil
2 eggs, beaten

200 g (7 oz) yellow onion, trimmed, peeled, cored and minced

20 g (³/₄ oz) spring onion, roots and coarse tops cut off, minced

300 g (11 oz) asparagus, coarse bottoms cut off, cut into 1-cm (¹/₂-in)-long batons

200 g (7 oz) unsalted tinned sockeye or Alaska salmon in water, drained

1 tbsp sake (sold for drinking, not cooking)

Pinch of sea salt (do not add if using salted tinned salmon)

¹/₂ tsp low-sodium soy sauce

Freshly ground black pepper

1 tbsp fresh chopped coriander leaves

750 g (1 lb 12 oz) cooked Japanese short-grain rice (white or brown) (see page 97)

· · · · · · · · · · · · · ·

1. Place a wok (or a large frying pan with good heat conductivity) over a high heat. Add 1 tbsp of the oil and swirl it around to coat the interior of the wok. When the oil begins to simmer, add the beaten eggs; they will immediately begin to puff in the middle and bubble around the edges.

2. Fry the eggs for 2 minutes on medium heat, or until the centre portion is no longer runny. Turn the omelette and fry for 1 more minute. Transfer to a plate. When the omelette is cool enough to handle, tear it into bite-size pieces.

3. Add the remaining 2 tbsp of oil to the wok. When hot, add the onions and asparagus. Stir-fry for 2 minutes over medium-high heat. Add the sake, salt, soy sauce and a couple of grinds of pepper. Reduce the heat to medium and add the salmon, cooked rice, the bits of torn omelette and the chopped coriander leaves. With a spatula, crumble the salmon.

4. Toss the ingredients in the wok and stir-fry for 3 minutes, or until the rice and salmon are hot. Serve in medium-size individual bowls.

VINEGARED SUSHI RICE

Makes 750 g (1 lb 12 oz)

370 g (13 oz) short-grain white rice
570 ml (20 fl oz) cold water
1 tbsp sake (sold for drinking, not cooking)

Vinegar mixture

2 tbsp brown rice vinegar
2 tsp sugar
1 tsp mirin
1 tsp salt

Cooker-top method

ingredients listed above

1. Wash the rice (unless you are using haiga-mai) according to the instructions for fluffy rice (see page 97).
2. To cook the rice, transfer the washed grains to a medium saucepan. Add the water and sake and leave the rice to soak for 20 minutes until plump. Cover the saucepan and bring the rice to the boil. Reduce the heat to low and gently simmer the rice for 15 minutes (longer for brown rice), or until all the liquid has evaporated. Turn off the heat and let the rice sit, covered, for 10 minutes.
3. Meanwhile, in a small saucepan, heat the ingredients for the vinegar mixture over medium heat, stirring until the sugar is dissolved, but do not boil the mixture.
4. Scoop the cooked rice into a wooden *sushi oke* (tub) with a

rice paddle. Taking care not to squish the rice grains, pour the vinegar mixture evenly over the rice and gently toss to mix. The rice is now ready for various sushi recipes.

Electric rice cooker method

ingredients listed on page 175

1. Wash the rice according to the instructions for fluffy rice (see page 97).
2. To cook the rice, transfer the washed grains to the cooking bowl of an electric rice cooker. Add enough cold water to the bowl, according to the machine's instructions, for 370 g (13 oz) of dry rice and then add the sake. Leave the rice to soak for 20 minutes until plump.
3. Plug in the rice cooker and push the On or Start button. When the rice has finished cooking, let it rest undisturbed for 10 minutes (do not open the lid).
4. Meanwhile, make the vinegar mixture (see the cooker-top method).
5. After the cooked rice has been sitting for 10 minutes, mix the rice and the vinegar mixture (see the cooker-top method).

TRI-COLOUR VEGETABLES OVER SUSHI RICE

Serves 2

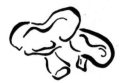

2 dried shiitake mushrooms

100 ml (4 fl oz) water

2 tbsp sake (sold for drinking, not cooking)

1 tbsp mirin

2 tbsp soya

Pinch of sea salt

200 g (7 oz) carrots, trimmed and sliced into 3-mm (⅛-in)
   thickness rounds
10 asparagus (about 150 g/5 ½ oz), woody stem ends snapped off,
   and each spear cut diagonally into 2- to 3-cm (approx. 1-in)
   pieces. Set aside several asparagus tips for the garnish
100 g (3 ½ oz) celery, trimmed and cut into 3-mm thick slices
50 g (1 ¾ oz) leek, cut into 3-mm thick slices
750 g (1 lb 12 oz) cooked vinegared sushi rice (see page 175)
10 g (½ oz) toasted & ground white sesame seeds (see page 171)
2 small sprigs of mitsuba

• • • • • • • • • • • • • •

1. Place the shiitake mushrooms in a small bowl and add 100 ml
    (4 fl oz) of water. Leave to soak for 20 minutes. Remove the
    mushroom soaking water into a small bowl, blend in the soy
    sauce, the mirin, the sake and the salt.

2. Drain the mushrooms, squeeze gently to remove excess
    water. Cut off the stems. Cut each cap into thin slices.

3. In a medium saucepan, add the sliced carrots, asparagus,
    celery, leek and mushroom cap slices and the shiitake dashi
    mixture. Simmer over medium heat for 15 minutes, or until
    the carrots are cooked through.

4. Lay out 2 bowls. Fill each one with 375 g (13 oz) of vinegared
    sushi rice and artistically arrange even portions of the simmered
    vegetables over the top. Garnish each serving with a sprinkling
    of the sesame seeds, asparagus tips and 1 sprig of mitsuba.

SEAFOOD MEDLEY OVER SUSHI RICE

Serves 2

....

100 g (3 ½ oz) mange tout
250 g (9 oz) Alaska wild salmon fillet
8 jumbo prawns, shelled and de-veined

1 tbsp sake (sold for drinking, not cooking)
1 tbsp low-sodium soy sauce
1 tsp mirin
Pinch of sea salt
2 large eggs
1 tbsp dashi
Tiny pinch of salt
Freshly ground black pepper
2 tsp rapeseed oil
750 g (1 lb 12 oz) cooked vinegared sushi rice (see page 175)
2 tbsp shredded nori sea vegetables
2 sprigs of mitsuba
Wasabi, optional, to use at the table

....

1. Bring a small saucepan of water to the boil. Add the mange tout and cook over a medium-high heat for 1–2 minutes, or until crisp yet tender. Drain and refresh under cold water. Drain and slice the mange tout into julienne strips. Set aside.

2. To cook the seafood, place the fish fillet and prawns in a shallow dish and season both sides with sake, soy sauce, mirin and salt. Heat a large non-stick grill pan under a high heat. When hot, add the seasoned fish and prawns and grill under a medium heat for 4 minutes.

3. Turn and grill the seafood for 2 more minutes, or until the centre of the fillet flakes when prodded with a sharp knife. Transfer the salmon fillet to a cutting board and slice it into 8 equal pieces.

4. While the fish is grilling, in a small bowl place the eggs, dashi and salt, and a little freshly ground black pepper, and whisk until well mixed.

5. Place a large non-stick frying pan over medium heat. Add 1 tbsp of oil and swirl the pan until the surface is evenly coated. Pour the egg mixture into the frying pan. Tilt the pan to coat the surface evenly with the egg. Cook for 2 minutes, or until the egg begins to pucker around the edges and the bottom of the egg disc is golden brown.

6. Carefully turn the egg disc over with a spatula and fry the other side for 2 minutes, or until the bottom is golden brown. Transfer the egg disc to a cutting board and slice it into julienne strips. Set aside.

7. Lay out 2 bowls. Fill each one with 375 g (13 oz) of vinegared sushi rice and artistically arrange even portions of seafood, eggs and mange tout over the top. Garnish each serving with a sprinkling of shredded nori sea vegetable and 1 sprig of mitsuba.

SOUPS

CAULIFLOWER–NAPA CABBAGE 'EAST-MEETS -WEST' SOUP
....

Serves 4
....

1 tbsp rapeseed oil

1 medium-size yellow onion, trimmed, peeled and finely chopped (about 190 g/6 ¹/₂ oz)

3 medium-size carrots, trimmed and diagonally sliced (about 300 g/11 oz)

1 tsp sake (sold for drinking, not cooking)

370 g (13 oz) cauliflower (purple, if available), stemmed and cut into bite-size chunks

500 g (1 lb) napa cabbage, cut into bite-size pieces, separating tender leaves and thick white bottom portions

1 leek, root and dark green portions removed, diagonally sliced

900 ml (1 ¹/₂ pints) dashi (see recipe page 168)

10 sprigs fresh coriander, chopped

....

1. Heat the oil in a medium saucepan over a medium-high heat. Stir in the onion and lower the heat to medium. When the onion is translucent, add the carrots and cauliflower and stir-fry until crisp yet tender.

2. Add the sake, thick white bottom portions of napa, leek and dashi. Simmer over medium heat until tender, stirring occasionally. Add the tender leaves of napa and coriander and simmer for a few more minutes. Serve in deep soup bowls.

MISO SOUP WITH EXTRA FIRM TOFU & SPRING ONIONS

....

Serves 2

....

125 g (4 oz) extra firm tofu

750 ml (1 ¼ pint) dashi (see page 168)

1 spring onion, root and rough portion of the top cut off, and thinly
  sliced

1 tbsp lower-sodium red or white miso (or use a combination of both)

....

1. Place the tofu in a colander or strainer and gently rinse under
   cold water. Drain and cut the tofu into small, diced pieces.
2. Place the dashi in a medium saucepan and bring the mixture
   to the boil. Stir in the spring onions and tofu and bring the
   mixture back to the boil. Reduce the heat to medium and
   cook for 2 minutes, or until the onions are tender.
3. Gently whisk in the miso and turn off the heat. Ladle the soup
   into two small bowls.

MISO SOUP WITH CLAMS & MITSUBA

Serves 2

6 manila clams

30 g (1 oz) sea salt

1.2 litres (2 pints) cold water

1 tbsp lower-sodium red or white miso (or use a combination of both)

2 sprigs of mitsuba, stem knotted

1. Scrub the clams under cold water to eliminate any dirt from the shells, then rinse the clams in several changes of water, until the water runs clear. To get rid of any grit inside the shells, dissolve the salt in 450 ml (¾ pint)of the cold water and soak the clams in the salt solution in the refrigerator for 20 minutes. Drain and then rinse.

2. Place the remaining 750 ml (1¼ pint) of cold water in a medium saucepan. Add the clams. Bring the liquid to the boil, then add the sake. Skim the foam from the surface of the liquid with a ladle. As soon as the clams open, which should be only a few minutes after the water comes to the boil, they are cooked.

3. Gently whisk in the miso until dissolved then turn off the heat. Lay out two small soup bowls. Using kitchen tongs, arrange three clams and a mitsuba sprig in each bowl. Ladle the soup over the clams and garnish with spring onions. Place a bowl in the centre of the table for the discarded shells.

MISO SOUP WITH WAKAME SEA VEGETABLE & SPRING ONIONS

Serves 2

....

2 g (2 tbsp) dried wakame sea vegetable

30 g (1 oz) spring onions, root and rough portion of the top cut off, and thinly sliced

750 ml (1¼ pint) dashi (see page 168)

1 tbsp lower-sodium red or white miso (or use a combination of both)

....

1. In a medium bowl, soak the wakame in 450 ml (¾ pint) water for about 15 minutes, or until expanded and tender. Drain and cut into 3-cm (1-in) ribbons.

2. Place the dashi in a medium saucepan and bring the mixture to the boil. Stir in the wakame and spring onions and bring the mixture back to the boil. Reduce the heat to medium and cook for 2 minutes, or until the onions are tender.

3. Gently whisk in the miso and turn off the heat. Ladle the soup into two small soup bowls.

SALADS

ASPARAGUS SALAD WITH WHITE SESAME DRESSING
· · · · · · · · · · · · · ·

Serves 2
· · · · · · · · · · · · ·

100 g (3 ¹/₂ oz) fresh asparagus, rinsed and coarse bottom of stems
    removed (you can substitute asparagus with French beans,
    cauliflower, kale or spinach)
10 ml (¹/₂ oz) white sesame seed dressing (see page 172)
· · · · · · · · · · · · · ·

1. Bring a large saucepan of water to the boil. Turn down to medium-high heat, add the asparagus and cook for 3 minutes, or until just crisp yet tender and bright green (for leafy vegetables like kale and spinach, cooking time is shorter).
2. Drain and refresh under cold water and dry with paper towels (for leafy vegetables, squeeze the liquid and wrap in paper towels). Cut the asparagus stems diagonally into 3-cm (1-in) slices and place in a small bowl. Pour the white sesame seed dressing over the asparagus and toss well to combine.

RADISH SALAD
· ·

Serves 2
· · · · · · · · · · · · ·

100 g (3¹/₂ oz) radishes (about five), trimmed and sliced into 2 mm
    (¹/₈ in) thin rounds
Pinch of sea salt
50 ml (2 fl oz) traditional Japanese vinaigrette (see page 170)
1 tsp fresh chopped purple basil leaves
· · · · · · · · · · · · · ·

In a bowl, sprinkle the salt over the sliced radish, mix, and squeeze the liquid out of the radish. Pour the vinaigrette over the radish and toss to mix well. Serve cool in individual small bowls and garnish with the chopped basil leaves.

CHILLED CUCUMBER SALAD

Serves 2

Pinch of sea salt
200 g (7 oz) chilled seedless cucumbers
50 ml (1³/₄ fl oz) chilled creamy tofu sauce (see page 171)

Rub the salt onto the cucumber skin, trim and slice the cucumbers diagonally 5 mm (¼ in) thick and squeeze any liquid out of the sliced cucumbers. Just before serving, in a small bowl, toss the cucumbers and creamy tofu sauce. Serve cool on individual salad plates.

SUMMER RIPE TOMATO & TOFU SALAD

Serves 2

200 g (7 oz) firm tofu
2 ripe medium-size chilled tomatoes, cored and sliced into 1 cm
     (¹/₂ in) thick rounds
Extra-virgin olive oil
Sea salt and freshly ground black pepper to taste
1 tsp chopped basil leaves

1. Wrap the tofu in two layers of paper towel or muslin and place in a microwave-safe container. Microwave for 3 minutes.
2. Unwrap and drain the tofu. Slice into 1 cm (½ in) thick slices, cover and chill in a fridge.
3. On a serving platter, layer the tomato and the chilled tofu slices alternately. Drizzle the oil, sprinkle on the salt, the pepper and the basil.

EDAMAME MESCLUN SALAD
••

Serves 2
••••••••••••••

150 g (5½ oz) frozen shelled edamame soya beans
150 g (5½ oz) mesclun (mixed leaves)
1 tsp fresh chopped basil leaves
2 whole basil leaves
100 ml (4 fl oz) sesame oil salad dressing (see page 170)
••••••••••••••••

1. Bring a medium saucepan of water to the boil, add the edamame and simmer for about 5 minutes, or until crispy yet tender. Drain well.
2. Combine the cooked edamame, leaves and basil in a salad bowl. Gently toss to mix. Pour the dressing over the salad and gently toss to mix.
3. Lay out 2 salad plates. Arrange a portion of salad on each plate and garnish with a basil leaf.

BEETROOT LEAVES SALAD WITH LEMON DRESSING

Serves 2

300 g (11 oz) beetroot leaves, stems removed, thoroughly rinsed
   (stems can be saved and used for another dish such as stir-fry
   or soup)
Juice of 1 lemon (2 ½ tbsp)
1 tsp granulated sugar
Pinch of sea salt

1. Bring a large saucepan of water to the boil. Add the beetroot leaves and cook over a medium-high heat for 30 seconds. Drain and refresh under cold water.
2. Gently squeeze the beetroot leaves to remove excess water. Tightly wrap the leaves in a paper towel or muslin and store in a refrigerator.
3. Meanwhile blend together the lemon juice, sugar and a generous pinch of salt in a small bowl until the sugar dissolves.
4. Unwrap the beetroot leaves and cut into 3 cm (1-in) chunks, squeeze out any excess water and add to the lemon dressing. Toss well to combine. Serve immediately.

SEARED JUMBO PRAWNS ON A BED OF MESCLUN SALAD

Serves 2

10 prawns
1 tbsp sake (sold for drinking, not cooking)
Pinch of sea salt and freshly ground black pepper
150 g (5½ oz) mesclun salad (mixed leaves)
100 ml (4 fl oz) sesame oil salad dressing (see page 170)
4 lemon wedges
2 coriander sprigs

1. De-vein each prawn and peel off the shell, except the last shell segment closest to the tail and the tail itself (or ask your fishmonger to do it for you). Sprinkle the sake, salt and pepper over them on both sides.
2. Sear the prawns under a grill for 2 minutes each side, or until orange and cooked.
3. In a large bowl, pour the dressing over the salad and gently toss to mix.
4. Lay out two salad plates. Arrange a portion of salad on each plate and garnish with five prawns, two lemon wedges and a coriander sprig.

VEGETABLE DISHES

SAUTÉED BEETROOTS

Serves 2

1 tbsp rapeseed oil
3 small beetroots, trimmed and sliced into 5-mm ($^{1}/_{4}$-in) thick
    rounds (about 250 g/9 oz)
1 tsp sake (sold for drinking, not cooking)

1. Heat a large frying pan and add the oil. When the oil is hot,
    add the beetroot, sauté on medium-high, add the sake,
    continue to sauté until the beetroots are crisp on the outside
    and all the liquid has evaporated from the pan (about
    5 minutes).
2. Transfer the beetroots to a rack lined with a double layer of
    paper towel to drain excess oil. Serve hot.

STEAMED VEGGIES WITH GINGER SOY SAUCE

Serves 2

150 g ($5^{1}/_{2}$ oz) courgettes, trimmed and sliced
150 g ($5^{1}/_{2}$ oz) yellow courgettes, trimmed and sliced
100 g ($3^{1}/_{2}$ oz) potato, trimmed and quartered
100 g ($3^{1}/_{2}$ oz) green pepper, thickly sliced
1 small yellow onion, trimmed, peeled, cored and quartered
    (100 g/$3^{1}/_{2}$ oz)

. . . .

10 g (½ oz) zested ginger root, to add at the table
Low-sodium soy sauce, to add at the table

. . . .

In a steamer, boil the water on a high heat. Place the vegetables in the steamer and cook for 20 minutes on medium heat, or until the potatoes are cooked through and other vegetables are crisp yet tender. Let each diner season the vegetables with the ginger root and soy sauce.

LIGHTLY SAUTÉED FIVE COLOUR VEGGIES & TOFU CHUNKS: BROCCOLI, CARROT, ONION, YELLOW COURGETTE & RED BELL PEPPER

. . . .

Serves 2

. . . .

100 g (3½ oz) extra-firm tofu
1 medium-size yellow onion, trimmed, peeled and sliced into bite-size pieces (200 g/7 oz)
2 cloves garlic, trimmed and minced
50 g (1¾ oz) shallots, trimmed and minced
¼ head of broccoli florets, coarse bottom cut off (about 200 g)
2 medium carrots, trimmed and sliced diagonally 1 cm (½ in) thick (about 200 g/7 oz)
1 yellow courgette, trimmed and sliced diagonally 1 cm (½ in) thick (about 250 g/9 oz)
1 red bell pepper, seeded and sliced into bite sizes (about 240 g/8 ½ oz)
1 tbsp rapeseed oil
60 ml (2 fl oz) water
1 tbsp sake (sold for drinking, not cooking)
1 tbsp low-sodium soy sauce

Pinch of sea salt
Pinch of freshly ground black pepper, to taste
100 g (3 ½ oz) fresh ginger, grated
2 sprigs of coriander

. . . .

1. Rinse the tofu under cold water. Drain, cut into 2-cm (1-in) cubes and set aside.
2. Heat the oil in a wok or large sauté pan over a high heat. Add the onion, garlic, shallots and carrots and stir-fry for 3 minutes on a medium-high heat. Add the broccoli and carrots and stir-fry for 3 minutes.
3. Stir in the water, sake, soy sauce and salt and cook for 3 minutes. Add the yellow courgette, salt and pepper. Continue stir-frying the vegetables for 3 more minutes, or until the carrots are cooked through.
4. Add the tofu, red pepper and ginger, toss to mix and stir-fry for 2 minutes, or until most (if not all) of the seasoning liquid has evaporated.
5. Transfer to a large serving bowl and garnish with coriander leaves. Let each diner serve modest portions on an individual plate.

GRILLED PORTABELLO MUSHROOM OPEN SANDWICH WITH CREAMY TOFU SAUCE

. . . .

Serves 2

. . . .

Two portabello (large, flat) mushroom caps
    (about 10 cm/4 in diameter)
1 medium-size yellow onion, trimmed, peeled and sliced
    (about 200 g)
2 slices of multi-grain bread

2 tbsp creamy tofu sauce (see page 171)
Low-sodium stone-ground mustard, optional
10 rocket leaves, rinsed and dried
2 cherry tomatoes, trimmed and quartered

. . . .

1.   Pre-heat a non-stick grill on medium-high. Grill the mushroom caps and onion for 3 minutes each side, or until slightly browned.
2.   Lay out 2 medium plates. Place a slice of bread on each plate and spread the tofu sauce and mustard on the bread. Layer the rocket leaves, mushroom cap and onion on the bread. Garnish each plate with a quartered tomato.

KINPIRA CARROTS WITH HOT CHILLI PEPPERS

Serves 4

. . . .

1 tbsp rapeseed oil
2 dried Japanese red peppers, (or Thai chilli, Santaka or Szechuan peppers)
260 g (9 oz) carrot, cut into matchstick-size slivers
1 tbsp sake (sold for drinking, not cooking)
1 tbsp reduced-sodium soy sauce
2 tsp mirin
1 tsp granulated sugar
1 tsp toasted and ground sesame seeds

. . . .

1.   Heat the oil in a medium-size frying pan over a medium-high heat. Add the red peppers and sauté for 30 seconds. Add the carrot and sauté until tender, about 3 minutes.
2.   Reduce the heat to low and add the sake, soy sauce, mirin and

sugar. Stir the carrots for 1 minute more to allow them to absorb the sauce.

3. Remove and discard the red peppers, arrange the vegetables in a mound in the centre of a serving bowl and garnish with the sesame seeds.

AUBERGINES & GREEN PEPPERS WITH RED MISO DRESSING

••••••••••••••••••••••

Serves 4

••••••••••••••

450 g (1 lb) Japanese aubergines (or Italian aubergines), stem caps
    cut off, peeled and cut into bite-size pieces
2 tbsp mirin
2 tbsp lower-sodium red miso
2 tsp granulated sugar
1 tsp sake (sold for drinking, not cooking)
225 ml (8 fl oz) rapeseed oil
1 green pepper, cored, seeded and cut into bite-size pieces
1 tsp toasted & ground white sesame seeds (see page 171)
½ tsp toasted sesame oil

••••••••••••••

1. Soak the aubergine pieces in a bowl of water for a few minutes. Drain and thoroughly wipe off excess water with kitchen towel. In a small bowl, blend the mirin, miso, sugar and sake. Set aside.

2. Heat the oil in a wok or large deep frying pan over a medium heat until it reaches 180°C/350°F. If you don't have a cooking thermometer, test the oil with a tiny square of fresh bread. If the bread rises and immediately turns golden, then the oil is hot enough.

3. Carefully slip the aubergine pieces into the oil. Fry for

3 minutes, adjusting the heat as necessary to keep the oil temperature at around 180°C/350°F. Rotate and fry the aubergine on all sides, for 1 to 2 minutes more, or until the flesh is soft. Test for doneness by piercing the flesh with a wooden skewer: you should be able to slide it easily all the way through.

4. Transfer the aubergine pieces to a rack lined with a double layer of paper towel to drain. Pour off the oil from the wok into a metal container (to discard or use on another occasion).

5. The wok will still be coated with a small amount of oil. Place the wok over a medium-high heat and add the pepper. Stir-fry for 2 minutes, or until the pepper is bright green. Add the aubergine pieces and the miso mixture, and gently toss the vegetables to coat with the sauce.

6. Transfer to a serving dish and garnish with the toasted and ground sesame seeds and sesame oil.

VEGETABLE GYOZA DUMPLINGS

Serves 4

150 g (5 1/2 oz) finely chopped cabbage

5 fresh shiitake mushrooms, stems removed and caps minced

1/2 bunch nira (Chinese chives or garlic chives) finely chopped (or 45 g (1 1/2 oz) finely chopped regular chives or shallots)

2 spring onions, roots and coarse top cut off, minced

Pinch of sea salt and freshly ground black pepper

24 round gyoza dumpling wrappers (find them in supermarkets or Asian grocery stores)

2 tbsp rapeseed oil

225 ml (8 fl oz) water

Dipping sauce

•••••••••••••

50 ml (2 fl oz) low-sodium soy sauce

50 ml (2 fl oz) brown rice vinegar

$^{1}/_{2}$ tsp sesame oil

Shichimi togarashi, or crushed hot pepper oil, to use at the table
(optional)

Unsalted stone-ground mustard, to use at the table (optional)

•••••••••••••

1. Place the cabbage, mushrooms, chives and spring onions in a
    large bowl. Season with several generous pinches of salt and
    a little black pepper. Use your hands to blend the ingredients
    together.

2. For each dumpling, place 2 tsp of filling in the centre of a
    gyoza wrapper.

3. Fill a small bowl with cold water. Lightly wet one finger in the
    water and trace around the inside of the gyoza wrapper,
    which will make it sticky enough to seal.

4. Fold the wrapper in half, with the edge on top, and gently
    press the edges from right to left to seal the dumpling,
    while pinching and folding every 6 mm (¼ in) of the edge
    facing you to make a zigzag pattern. Place the completed
    dumplings on a foil-lined baking sheet with the crimped
    side up.

5. To make the dipping sauce, mix the soy sauce, vinegar and oil
    in a small bowl or jar. Set aside until serving time.

6. Place a large, deep frying pan over a high heat and add 2
    tbsp of oil. When hot, reduce the heat to medium-low and
    add the dumplings, crimped side up. Cook, uncovered,
    until lightly browned on the bottom, about 4 minutes. (No
    need to turn.)

7. Pour the water into the frying pan. Cover with a lid and
    steam-cook the dumplings over a medium heat for 8–10
    minutes, adding a tad more water as necessary, until the tops
    of the dumplings are translucent and all the water has

evaporated. (If tops turn translucent before the water has evaporated, remove cover and continue cooking until water has gone.)

8. Transfer six dumplings to each serving plate, golden sides uppermost. Lay out four small plates to hold dipping sauce and serve.

Extra-healthy variation

STEAMED DUMPLINGS

Instead of frying the dumplings, steam them in a steamer for 15 minutes, or until the filling is cooked through. Serve with the same dipping sauce.

SIMMERED DAIKON & TOFU

Serves 4

400 g (14 oz) fresh daikon (Japanese giant white radish, see page 217, or use ordinary radish), cut into bite-size pieces
590 ml (1 pint) dashi (see recipe page 168)
250 g (9 oz) firm tofu, cut into bite-size cubes
1 tsp sea salt
1 tsp granulated sugar, or natural cane sugar
2 tsp sake (sold for drinking, not cooking)
1 tsp low-sodium soy sauce

1. Place the daikon and dashi in a medium saucepan over a medium-high heat and bring to the boil. Reduce the heat to medium-low and stir in the salt, sugar, sake and soy sauce.

2. Place a drop-lid (or a piece of aluminium foil cut to a slightly smaller diameter than the saucepan, see page 232) over the ingredients and simmer, stirring occasionally,

until the daikon have absorbed ⅔ of the liquid (about 50 minutes).

3. Add the tofu and simmer until the daikon and tofu have absorbed almost all the liquid (about 10 minutes longer). Transfer to a serving bowl.

FISH DISHES

SARDINES & CHERRY TOMATOES

Serves 2

1 tbsp rapeseed oil
1 tin (about 120 g/4 oz) sardines in water
10 cherry tomatoes, trimmed and cut in half lengthways
Sea salt and freshly ground black pepper, to taste
2 tsp chopped spring onions
$^1/_2$ lemon, cut into two $^1/_4$ wedges

1. Add the oil to a small non-stick frying pan and heat on high. When the oil is hot, bring the heat down to medium-high, add the sardines, sprinkle a pinch of salt and black pepper over the fish and cook for 2 minutes. Add the tomatoes and spring onions and gently sauté for 2 minutes.
2. Lay out two plates. Arrange equal portions of the sardines, tomatoes and spring onions on each plate and garnish with a lemon wedge. Serve hot. Let each diner squeeze the lemon juice over the fish.

SIMMERED BASS IN MILD TERIYAKI SAUCE

Serves 2

2 fillets of bass (60 g/2 oz each)
2 tbsp sake (sold for drinking, not cooking)
1 tbsp mirin
2 tbsp low-sodium soy sauce
Pinch of salt

30 ml (1 1/2 tbsp) water
Garnish: 1 tbsp minced spring onions

· · · · · · · · · · · · · ·

1. Lay the bass fillets in a small saucepan. Add the sake, mirin, soy sauce, salt and water to the pan and simmer over a medium heat for 4 minutes. Turn the fish and simmer for 2 minutes, or until cooked through.
2. Transfer the fish to individual shallow bowls and spoon the sauce over the fish. Garnish with the minced spring onions.

GRILLED MACKEREL

Serves 2

· · · · · · · · · · · · · ·

2 fillets of mackerel (120 g/4 oz each)
2 tsp salt
2 tbsp sake (sold for drinking, not cooking)
120g (4 oz) finely grated daikon (Japanese giant white radish, see page 217, or use ordinary radish), excess liquid drained off
Low-sodium soy sauce, to use at the table

· · · · · · · · · · · · · ·

1. Place the mackerel on a mesh tray, rub the salt over the fish and let moisture drain off the fish. Pat the fish with paper towel to remove excess moisture. Sprinkle sake over the fish.
2. Preheat a non-stick grill on medium-high. Pop in the fish fillets and grill for 5–7 minutes. Turn and grill the fillets for 5 more minutes, or until the centre of one fish flakes when prodded with a sharp knife.
3. Transfer the fish to individual plates and place a small amount of grated daikon (or radish) next to the fillet. Let each diner drizzle a drop or two of soy sauce over the daikon to flavour, then put the grated daikon and soya mixture on to a piece of fish.

GRILLED SALMON, BROCCOLI & ONIONS OVER FLUFFY RICE

••••••••••••••••••••••••••••

Serves 2

••••••••••••••••

1 tbsp rapeseed oil

¹/₂ large yellow onion, peeled, halved and cut into thin crescents
    (150 g/5 oz)

200 g (7 oz) broccoli florets, steamed

2 tsp sake (sold for drinking, not cooking)

1 tsp mirin

1 tsp low-sodium soy sauce

2 tbsp water

Pinch of sea salt and freshly ground black pepper

2 salmon fillets (115 g/4 oz each)

1 tbsp sake (sold for drinking, not cooking)

2 tbsp shredded Nori sea vegetables

Pinch of salt

750 g (1 lb 12 oz) cooked rice (see page 97)

120g (4 oz) finely grated daikon (Japanese giant white radish, see
    page 217, or use ordinary radish), excess liquid drained off

A few drops of low-sodium soy sauce

2 sprigs of mitsuba (Japanese parsley)

••••••••••••••••

1. Heat the oil in a wok or medium sauté pan over a high heat. Add
    the onion and stir-fry for 5 minutes on medium. Add the broccoli
    and cook for 3 minutes, until bright green and crisp yet tender.

2. Stir in the sake, the mirin, the soy sauce, the water, the salt
    and the pepper and simmer for 3 more minutes. Turn off the
    heat and set aside.

3. Place the fish fillets in a shallow dish and season both sides
    with the sake and a pinch of salt. Preheat the grill to medium-
    high. Place the salmon fillets on a rack in a grilling pan, and
    grill under a medium heat for 5–7 minutes. Turn and grill the

salmon for 5 more minutes, or until the centre of one fillet flakes when prodded with a sharp knife.

4. Lay out two bowls. Fill each one with 375 g (13 oz) of hot cooked rice, sprinkle the nori sea vegetables and arrange the stir-fried vegetables and the grilled salmon. Garnish each serving with a small amount of grated daikon and a sprig of parsley. Let each diner drizzle a couple of drops of soy sauce over the daikon to flavour. To eat, put some grated daikon and soya onto a piece of fish.

SCRAMBLED TOFU WITH SALMON

Serves 2

200 g (7 oz) firm tofu
1 tbsp rapeseed oil
50 g (1 ¹/₄ oz) tinned Alaska salmon in water, drained
Salt and freshly ground black pepper, to taste
3 spring onions, white and light green parts minced

1. Wrap the tofu in two layers of paper towel or muslin, place in a microwave-safe container and microwave for 3 minutes.
2. In a medium pan, heat the oil. When the oil is hot, reduce the heat to medium, add the tofu and break it up into random chunks with a spoon or spatula.
3. Add the salmon and break it up into random chunks, combining them with the tofu chunks. Sprinkle over the salt and black pepper. Turn off the heat.
4. Lay out two small plates, arrange the tofu salmon on each and garnish with the minced spring onions. Serve hot.

WHITE FISH, FIRM TOFU, LEEKS, CARROTS, STRING BEANS IN HEARTY ONE POT DISH WITH LIME JUICE

Serves 2

260 g (9 oz) of your choice white fish fillet (e.g. cod, catfish, tilapia), skinned and boned

1 tbsp sake (sold for drinking, not cooking)

Pinch of sea salt

200 ml (7 fl oz) dashi (see page 168)

1 tbsp sake (sold for drinking, not cooking)

1 tbsp low-sodium soy sauce

50 g (1³/₄ oz) carrot, trimmed and diagonally cut into 5 mm (¹/₄ in) thick, 3–5 cm (1–2 in) long oval slices

50 g (1³/₄ oz) leeks, cut into 5 cm (2 in) long julienne strips

150 g (5¹/₂ oz) firm tofu, water drained and cut into small cubes

50 g (1³/₄ oz) string beans (about 10), trimmed and cut into 5 cm (2 in) long strips

¹/₂ lime (or yuzu) juice, or 25 ml (1 tbsp) (see page 231)

1. Place the fish fillet on a tray and sprinkle sake over the fish. Slice the fillet into 8 pieces.
2. In a medium casserole, combine the dashi, sake, soy sauce, add the carrot and leek and simmer for 3 minutes on medium. Add the tofu, string beans and white fish, and simmer for another 5 minutes, or until the fish is cooked through, skimming the foam on the broth surface with a ladle.
3. Lay out two bowls. Ladle even portions of the fish and vegetable mixture and spoon the sauce over the mixture. Drizzle the lime (or yuzu) juice to taste.

Japan Diet Short-cut

A Japanese grocery store often carries yuzu citrus juice in a bottle. Look for it in the sauce section.

MEAT DISHES

JAPANESE COUNTRY STYLE SIMMERED CHICKEN, BROCCOLI & CARROT

Serves 2

• • • • • • • • • • • • • •

100 g (3 ½ oz) carrot, trimmed, cut into 5 cm (2 in) long, 1 cm (½ in) wide sticks

1 bunch baby broccoli (200 g/7 oz), stems peeled and florets cut off and set aside

560 ml (20 fl oz) dashi (see page 168)

1 tbsp low-sodium soy sauce

1 tsp sake (sold for drinking, not cooking)

250 g (9 oz) chicken breast, boned and skinned, sliced into bite-size chunks

Several lime peels

• • • • • • • • • • • • • •

1. Bring a medium saucepan of water to the boil. Add the carrots and simmer for 4 minutes on medium-high, or until crisp yet tender. Take the carrots out of the saucepan, run under cold water and drain. Set aside.

2. In the same cooking water, add the broccoli stems and simmer for 2 minutes, or until crisp yet tender. Take the broccoli stems out of the saucepan, run under cold water and drain. Set aside.

3. In the same cooking water, add the broccoli florets and simmer for 1 minute, or until bright green and crisp yet tender. Take the florets out of the saucepan, run under cold water and drain. Set aside.

4. In a medium saucepan, heat the cooking stock, soy sauce and sake. Add the chicken chunks and cook on medium heat, skimming the foam on the broth surface, until the chicken is cooked through (about 10 minutes).

5. Lay out two bowls. Arrange equal portions of the chicken chunks, carrot sticks, broccoli stems and florets in each bowl and spoon the hot broth over them. Garnish each serving with a couple of lime peels. Serve hot.

CHICKEN & EGGS (PARENT & CHILD) OVER FLUFFY RICE

Serves 4

4 large eggs
225 ml (8 fl oz) dashi (see page 168)
50 ml (2 fl oz) sake (sold for drinking, not cooking)
1 medium-size yellow onion, peeled, halved and cut into thin crescents
1 small leek, roots and rough portion of the top cut off, cleaned, rinsed and cut diagonally into thin slices
$^1/_2$ tsp low-sodium soy sauce
1 tsp granulated sugar
1 tsp salt
1 tsp mirin
225 g (8 oz) boneless, skinless chicken breasts, cut into bite-size pieces
1.5 kg (3 lb) hot cooked brown or white rice (see page 97)
4 sprigs of mitsuba (Japanese parsley, see page 221, or use Italian parsley or coriander)

1. Break the eggs into a medium bowl and whisk until just mixed. Place the dashi and sake in a medium saucepan over high heat. Add the onion and leek and bring the mixture to the boil. Reduce the heat to medium and simmer until the vegetables are tender (about 5 minutes).
2. Stir in the soy sauce, sugar, salt and mirin. Stir in the chicken pieces and cook for 3 minutes.

3. Pour the beaten eggs over the surface of the chicken mix, so that the egg forms a sort of 'cap'. Reduce the heat to low and cook the mixture for approximately 2 minutes, or until the egg and chicken are cooked through. Stir the mixture and turn off the heat.

4. Lay out 4 bowls. Fill each one with 375 g (13 oz) of hot cooked rice and ladle ¼ of the chicken-egg mixture over the top. Garnish each serving with a sprig of mitsuba.

BEEF, SWEET POTATO & ONION CASSEROLE – ONE POT DISH
••••••••••••••••••••••

Serves 2
•••••••••••••••

1 tbsp rapeseed oil

250 g (9 oz) lean minced sirloin beef

250 g (9 oz) medium-size sweet potato, cut to bite-size, 2 x 2 cm (³/₄ x ³/₄ in)

310 g (11 oz) large yellow onion, trimmed, peeled and sliced into 8 wedges

200 ml (7 fl oz) cold water

2 tbsp sake (sold for drinking, not cooking)

2 tbsp low-sodium soy sauce

Pinch of sea salt

•••••••••••••••

1. In a medium casserole, heat the oil and sauté the beef for 3 minutes on a medium-high heat. Remove the beef from the casserole and set aside.

2. In the same casserole, add the sweet potatoes and onions and sauté for 5 minutes on medium to medium-high heat.

3. Add the beef, the water, sake, soy sauce and salt to the casserole. Cover with a drop-lid (see page 232) and simmer

for 15 minutes on low-medium heat, or until the potatoes are cooked through, occasionally tossing the beef and vegetables to season evenly.

SOBA NOODLE DISHES

COOL SUMMER SOBA BUCKWHEAT NOODLE SALAD
· · · · · · · · · ·

Serves 2
· · · · · · · · · · · · · · ·

125 ml (4¹/₂ fl·oz) dashi (see page 168)
25 ml (1 fl oz) mirin
25 ml (1 fl oz) low-sodium soy sauce
200 g (7 oz) 100 per cent dry soba buckwheat noodles (see page 222)
2 large eggs
120 g (4 oz) firm tofu, water drained
2 tbsp rapeseed oil
1 medium-size yellow onion, trimmed, peeled and sliced into thin
　　crescents (about 190 g / 7 oz)
2 cloves of garlic, trimmed, peeled and minced
1 tbsp fresh chopped basil leaves

· · · · · · · · · · · · · · ·

1.　Combine the dashi, mirin and soy sauce in a small saucepan
　　over a high heat. Bring to the boil, turn off the heat and let
　　cool to room temperature. (Or, to speed up chilling, place the
　　cooled dipping sauce in a small metal bowl, nestle the small
　　metal bowl in a larger bowl half filled with ice and water, and
　　stir the sauce occasionally.)

2.　Place a large saucepan of water over a high heat and bring to
　　the boil. Add the soba and stir to prevent sticking. Cook the
　　soba, according to packet instructions, until just cooked
　　through. (Most soba cooks in 6 to 8 minutes, but test the
　　noodles as they boil.)

3.　Drain the soba when just past *al dente* and rinse in a colander
　　under cold water to remove any residual starch, and right

before serving, drench the noodles in ice water to tighten them, and drain.

4. In a food processor, mix the eggs and tofu, until smooth.

5. In a medium frying pan, heat 1 tbsp rapeseed oil. When the oil is hot, stir in the egg–tofu mixture. Fry the mixture for 3 minutes or until the bottom is golden. Turn the egg–tofu omelette over and fry for 2 more minutes, or until the bottom is golden brown. Transfer the omelette to a cutting board and slice into 8 pieces. Set aside.

6. In a frying pan, heat 1 tbsp rapeseed oil. When the oil is hot, add the onions and garlic, and sauté on medium heat for 3 minutes, or until the onions are translucent. Set aside.

7. Lay out two shallow bowls. Arrange equal amounts of noodles, top with eggs, onions, garlic and then pour the sauce over evenly. Garnish with the basil leaves.

Japan Diet Short-cut

You can buy ready-made dipping sauce at any Japanese market, or often at a gourmet grocer. The sauces are usually marked 'Dipping Sauce for Noodles – Ready to Use Soba Tsuyu' on the label.

BODY AND SOUL WARMING SOBA BUCKWHEAT NOODLES WITH SARDINE & SPINACH

Serves 4

500 g (1 lb) spinach, roots and coarse stems removed
900 ml (1 ½ pint) dashi (see page 168)
50 ml (2 fl oz) sake (sold for drinking, not cooking)
50 ml (2 fl oz) mirin
50 ml (2 fl oz) low-sodium soy sauce
1 tsp granulated sugar
1 tsp salt
450 g (1 lb) 100 per cent dry soba buckwheat noodles (see page 222)

120 g (4 oz) tinned de-skinned, de-boned sardine fillets in water (or
    vegetable oil), water drained
1 spring onion, roots and rough portion of the top cut off and thinly
    sliced
4 tiny sprigs of mitsuba (Japanese parsley, see page 221, or use
    Italian parsley or coriander)
Shichimi togarashi to be used at the table, optional (see page 227)
. . . .

1. Place the spinach in a large bowl filled with water; swish the
   leaves around to wash. If necessary, lift the spinach out of the
   water, empty the bowl and repeat the process until clean.

2. Bring a large saucepan of water to the boil. Reduce to a
   medium-high heat. Add the spinach and cook for 30
   seconds, or until just bright green and wilted. Drain and
   rinse under cold water. Gently squeeze the spinach to release
   excess water. Lay the spinach on a clean tea towel or muslin
   and gently roll up to absorb any remaining liquid. Set aside.

3. Place the dashi in a large saucepan over a high heat, stir in the
   sake, mirin, soy sauce, sugar and salt. Bring the mixture just
   to the boil, reduce heat to very low and keep warm.

4. Place a large saucepan of water over a high heat. Add the
   soba noodles and cook, stirring to prevent sticking, until
   just cooked through (about 6–8 minutes). When they are
   just past *al dente*, drain and rinse in a colander under cold
   water.

5. Unroll the spinach, squeeze out any excess water and cut it
   into 2.5-cm (1-in) pieces.

6. Bring the cooking broth back to the boil. Distribute four even
   portions of noodles among four large soup bowls. Lay a small
   mound of spinach and sardine fillet over the noodles and
   cover with the broth mixture. Garnish each serving with
   spring onions and a sprig of mitsuba. Season with shichimi
   togarashi, as desired.

SOBA BUCKWHEAT NOODLES WITH SHIITAKE, CRIMINI MUSHROOMS & GARLIC SAUCE

Serves 2

200 g (7 oz) 100 per cent dry soba buckwheat noodles
1 tbsp rapeseed oil
20 g (¾ oz) shallots, trimmed and minced
5 cloves garlic, trimmed and minced
250 g (9 oz) crimini mushrooms, cut into thin slices
100 ml (3½ fl oz) vegetable (shiitake) cooking stock (see page 167)
10 re-hydrated shiitake mushroom caps from the shiitake dashi
    (see page 186), cut into thin slices
1 tbsp sake (sold for drinking, not cooking)
¼ tsp low-sodium soy sauce
Pinch of sea salt
Freshly ground black pepper

1. Place a large saucepan of water over a high heat and bring to the boil. Add the soba and stir to prevent sticking. Cook according to packet instructions, until just cooked through. (Most soba cooks in 6 to 8 minutes, but test the noodles as they boil.)

2. Drain the soba when just past *al dente*, saving 100 ml (4 fl oz) of cooking water. Rinse in a colander under cold water to remove any residual starch.

3. Heat the oil in a wok or large sauté pan over a high heat. Add and stir-fry the minced shallots, garlic and crimini for 5 minutes on medium heat. Add the vegetable (shiitake) cooking stock and shiitake slices to the wok and simmer on medium-low, then blend them, along with the soba cooking liquid, sake, soy sauce, salt and pepper.

4. Toss to mix well and stir-fry for 5–7 minutes or until the broth has almost evaporated. Add the cooked soba noodles and toss gently to coat with the mushroom sauce. Serve immediately.

SOBA BUCKWHEAT NOODLES WITH SAUTÉED GREEN PEPPERS & STRING BEANS WITH GARLIC SOY SAUCE

....

Serves 2

....

200 g (7 oz) 100 per cent dry soba buckwheat noodles

1 tbsp rapeseed oil

20 g (³/₄ oz) shallot, trimmed and minced

5 cloves garlic, trimmed and minced

250 g (9 oz) green peppers, cored, seeded and sliced into vertical
    strips

150 g (5¹/₂ oz) string beans, trimmed and sliced diagonally into
    5-cm (2-in) strips

200 g (7 oz) leek cut into julienne strips

1 tbsp sake (sold for drinking, not cooking)

¹/₄ tsp low-sodium soy sauce

Pinch of sea salt

....

1. Place a large saucepan of water over a high heat and bring to the boil. Add the soba and stir to prevent sticking. Cook the soba, according to packet instructions, until just cooked through. (Most soba cooks for 6 to 8 minutes, but test the noodles as they boil.)

2. Drain when they are just past *al dente*, saving 100 ml (3½ fl oz) of cooking water. After draining, rinse the soba in a colander under cold water to remove any residual starch.

3. Heat the oil in a wok or large sauté pan over a high heat. Add and stir-fry the minced shallots and garlic for 5 minutes on medium heat. Add the green pepper slices, string beans and leeks to the wok and stir-fry for 3 minutes on medium heat, or until crisp yet tender. Then stir in the soba cooking liquid, sake, soy sauce, salt and pepper.

4. Toss to mix well and stir-fry for 5 minutes or until the broth has almost evaporated. Add the cooked soba noodles and toss gently to coat with the vegetable sauce. Serve immediately.

SNACKS

BANANAS ON TOASTED MULTI-GRAIN BREAD

Serves 2

2 bananas, peeled and cut diagonally into 1 cm (½ in) thick slices
4 slices of multi-grain bread

Toast the bread and layer the sliced bananas on top. Serve warm.

SLICED FUJI APPLES WITH CHEESES

Serves 4

Juice of ½ lemon
Cold water
2 Fuji apples (or any crispy, juicy, sweet apples)
100 g (3 ½ oz) each of 2 kinds of semi-hard strong cheese, such as
    Lord of The Hundreds Ewe's Milk, Gruyère and Comté
2 strawberries, cored, trimmed and sliced into quarters
A couple of mint leaves, or a small sprig of mint

1. In a medium-size bowl, mix the lemon juice with the cold water. Core and trim apple and slice into 5 mm (¼ in) thick crescents. Dip them in the water with lemon juice to avoid discoloration.
2. Drain the apples, pat dry with muslin and arrange on a serving platter.

3. Slice the cheeses into 5 mm (¼ in) thick rectangles, about the size of each apple slice, and layer them over the apple slices. Garnish with the strawberries and mint leaves.

HAND TO MOUTH – READY TO EAT FRUITS: STRAWBERRIES, CHERRIES, PLUMS, GRAPES, BANANAS
••••••••••••••

Any seasonal fresh fruits that are hassle free – such as strawberries, cherries, plums, grapes, bananas — no cutting, peeling, slicing required! Wash, dry and keep in a refrigerator until ready to enjoy.

VERY BERRIES: STRAWBERRIES, BLUEBERRIES & RASPBERRIES
•••••••••••••••••••••••••••••••••••••

Variety of berries, washed, chilled. When ready to eat, arrange them in pretty individual bowls.

SLICED SEASONAL FRUITS: APPLES, MANGOES, WATERMELONS, MELONS, PEARS, PEACHES, PLUMS
••••••••••••••••••••••••

Seasonal fruits washed, peeled, sliced and chilled in the fridge. When ready to eat, arrange a few pieces of the fruit on pretty individual plates.

STEAMED SWEET POTATOES

Serves 4

2 medium-size sweet potatoes, washed and cut into 3–4 cm
    (1–1³/₄ in) thick rounds (3 or 4 rounds from each)
Cold water

In a large steamer, add the water and the sweet potatoes and steam on medium-high heat for 20 minutes, or until the potatoes are done. Test by piercing the flesh with a wooden skewer: it should slide easily all the way through. Serve hot or at room temperature. Once cooled, will keep in an air-tight plastic bag in a refrigerator for up to three days.

TOKYO KITCHEN KEY INGREDIENTS

You can find most of the key ingredients, unique to Japanese home cooking, in the Asian food section of supermarkets, as well as in gourmet food shops and Japanese grocery stores. Here is an introduction to some basic Japanese cooking ingredients.

Bonito (fish) flakes (katsuobushi, hana-katsuo or kezuribushi)

A member of the mackerel family, bonito generally makes its appearance in Japanese cuisine not as a whole fish but as dried bonito fish flakes. These fish flakes, or *katsuo-bushi*, are an important ingredient in the Japanese kitchen. The larger fish flakes are used to make dashi, the essential cooking stock (see page 168), while the smaller flakes are used as a garnish for many dishes. Bonito flakes look like paper-thin curls of wood and range in colour from pinky beige to dark burgundy.

Although many Japanese people make their own fish flakes with a special bonito shaving implement, you can buy commercially shaved flakes in clear plastic bags. Large flakes for making dashi range in quantity from 28- to 450-g (1-oz to 1-lb) bags. The small fish flakes typically used for garnishes come in single-serving packets, usually five to a bag, with individual packets weighing anywhere from 15–25 g (½–1 oz). Bonito flakes have a mild, smoky, faintly sweet flavour. Although it's probably unlike anything you've encountered in Western cooking, it's a taste that's easy to acquire.

Daikon (white radish, white winter radish, Chinese white radish, Japanese giant white radish, or substitute ordinary radish)

Daikon is a large, white Japanese radish. It is quite juicy and has a fresh, sweet flavour and a mild bite. In her book *An American Taste of Japan*, Tokyo-based writer Elizabeth Andoh, the doyen of Western authorities on Japanese food, notes that daikon 'is perhaps the single most versatile vegetable in the Japanese repertoire; it can be grated or shredded and eaten raw; it can be steamed or braised and sauced or included in stews; it can be pickled or dried, too'.

I particularly like serving raw grated daikon with oily foods, since the spicy, wet radish provides an ideal counterpoint to deep-fried items and fatty fish, much the way that lemon does in Western cooking. Daikon also makes a tasty addition to miso soup – turning soft and almost sweet as it simmers in the savoury liquid.

Several varieties of fresh daikon are available in the West, including a green-necked version, which has a pale collar of green around the stem top area. When buying daikon, choose ones that are firm, not limp.

Edamame (fresh green soya beans)

Edamame are a popular accompaniment to cold beer in Japan. The fresh beans are available during the summer months at select shops and farmers' markets. If you can't find fresh edamame, the frozen ones, in their pods or without, make a fine, convenient substitute.

Japanese-style short-grain rice

Short-grain white rice is standard for Japanese home cooking. It is moister and stickier than medium- and long-grain rice. Short-grain brown rice, or genmai, is a high-fibre alternative.

Personally, I like to switch between white rice, brown rice and a third interesting option, haiga-mai (literally, rice-germ rice). This rice is partially polished, so it still contains the nutritious rice germ (usually removed in the milling process). I find haiga-mai tastes more nutty than polished white rice, but not quite as hearty as brown. Unlike the other rice types, haiga-mai should not be rinsed before cooking, in order to preserve the germ.

A premium variety of short-grain rice popular among Japanese is Koshihikari. Traditionally grown in Japan and sold under a number of different brand labels, this sweet, aromatic rice is now cultivated in the USA. In my opinion, American-grown short-grain rice is just as tasty as Japanese-grown rice. Store all rice in an airtight container in a cool, dry place, for up to a year.

. . . .

JAPANESE TEAS

Green teas

From sunrise to sundown, green tea flows like water in most Japanese homes and restaurants. And although the Japanese love coffee and black tea, they're crazy about their green tea.

It seems as if there's green tea brewing in my parents' dining room or kitchen all day long. When I'm there, my mother never asks, 'Would you like some tea?' She just keeps pouring it. Japanese green tea is gentle and clean-tasting, almost the opposite of coffee. It rejuvenates the soul, refreshes the palate and heals the body. Ancient priests and poets throughout China and Japan, as well as contemporary Western health experts, such as Andrew Weil, have sung the praises of this antioxidant superstar. Green tea is *never* served with sugar or milk, unless it becomes an ingredient for a dessert like green tea ice cream. There are many varieties of green tea. Here are descriptions of some of the most popular:

Sencha is the most popular green tea in a traditional Japanese home. It is grown in the sun.

Gyokuro, grown in the shade, is the finest, most expensive Japanese green tea.

Shin-cha, or new tea, is fresh harvest green tea, available in early summer.

Hojicha is roasted green tea leaves. When brewed, the tea, like the leaves themselves, is brown. It has a milder flavour than sencha and makes a great companion to fruits and other desserts.

Genmaicha is a mixture of green tea leaves and roasted brown rice. The rice adds a nutty, sweet grainy flavour to the tea.

Genmaimacha is a mixture of green tea leaves, roasted brown rice and powdered green tea. It has layers of flavour and is one of my favourites.

Mugicha (barley tea)

Mugicha (pronounced 'moo-gee-cha') is barley tea. Made cold, it is a healthy and delicious summertime drink, all year round. It's a great substitute for sweetened and carbonated beverages.

Tea leaves, tea bags and bottles

As with black tea, Japanese green tea is available in many forms: loose leaves, in tea bags and ready to drink in a bottle. With the exception of barley tea, I prefer to make my tea with loose leaves instead of bags because the leaves create a more fragrant and flavoursome brew.

....

Mirin (cooking wine)

Mirin is a sweet, golden cooking wine, made from glutinous rice, that has an alcohol content of about 14 per cent. It comes in a bottle and is used in many Japanese home-style recipes to add a bit of sweetness to simmered dishes, glazes and sauces.

Miso (fermented soya bean paste)

Miso is a thick, salty fermented soya bean paste that looks something like peanut butter and comes in refrigerated pouches or plastic tubs. It is made from crushed soya beans, salt, a fermenting agent and the addition of barley, rice or wheat. Depending upon which grain is added, the miso will vary tremendously in flavour, texture, aroma and colour. Miso can range in flavour from salty to sweet, in texture from smooth to slightly pebbly or chunky (with the addition of crushed grains or soya beans), in smell from delicate to pungent, and in colour from beige to golden yellow to brown.

In its many variations, miso is a staple of the Japanese kitchen and adds a savoury base note to soups, dressings, simmered dishes and stir-fries. So-called white miso is actually pale yellow and has a milder, sweeter flavour than other miso varieties. Because of its delicate nature, it's often used for dressings (particularly for vegetables) and in marinades for mild-tasting fish and seafood. So-called red miso, which appears rusty brown, is coarser and saltier than white. It works best in marinades and sauces for meats. The darkest brown version of red miso has the sharpest flavour and tastes best when added to simmered dishes containing oily fish or hearty meats. There are also mixed red-and-white versions of miso.

For miso soup as well as other dishes, many Japanese cooks keep two or three different kinds of miso in the refrigerator so that they can combine them to achieve their preferred taste. Like soy sauce, miso can sometimes be very high in salt, so look for lower-sodium or reduced-sodium miso by carefully reading the label. Restaurant chefs around the world have discovered the magic of miso and are using this bean paste to add a savoury flavour to boost a variety of dishes – not just Asian ones. Store miso in an airtight container in a refrigerator.

Mitsuba (Japanese parsley, trefoil; substitute Italian parsley and/or coriander)

Mitsuba, also known as trefoil or Japanese parsley, is a pretty garnish. It literally means 'three leaves' – as it looks. I have included it in several of the recipes in this book, though Italian parsley is fine to use in its place. A sprig of mitsuba, knotted and set afloat in clear soup, is exquisite.

Nira (Chinese chives, or garlic chives)

Nira is a member of the chive family and is also known as Chinese chives or garlic chives. The green leaves are flat, unlike the round chives commonly sold in the UK. I like their bold flavour – stronger than that of onions, but subtler than garlic. Substitute nira with shallots or chives. Nira also makes a great ingredient for stir-fry dishes.

....

NOODLES

Japan is awash with noodles. Family noodle shops dot the entire country from the northern island of Hokkaido to the Ryukyu Islands south of Kyushu. My mother loves to make a variety of noodle dishes and so do I. Some of the best meals I've eaten in Japan (aside from Mum's cooking, of course!) have come from nondescript mum-and-dad noodle shops. Whenever I go home to Tokyo, the first meal I have is almost always a bowl of noodles.

Japanese noodles fall into two major camps: those made with buckwheat flour (soba) and those made with white wheat flour (udon). Egg noodles, or ramen, are also very popular in Japan, mostly enjoyed as packet instant soups or in ramen specialist shops.

Soba (buckwheat) noodles

Soba is Japan's nutrition champion — a good source of protein, wholegrains, fibre and complex carbohydrates. Soba is the name for noodles made from buckwheat flour. They are thin, greyish brown and delightfully nutty tasting with a silky-smooth texture. They are served hot in soups, as well as cold with a tasty sweet soya dipping sauce.

Because buckwheat flour lacks gluten, the component in wheat flour that gives noodles their pleasant chewiness, most noodle makers add a little bit of starch to the dough. Some soba manufacturers add too much starch (in the form of white wheat flour or yam flour) – mainly to cut costs, since buckwheat flour costs more than other flours. The result is an inferior soba noodle that lacks the distinctive earthy flavour. Look for noodles that are as close to 100 per cent buckwheat as possible.

Soba noodles made exclusively from buckwheat flour are really worth the search. Brands like Clearspring, for example, are sold online. Among soba purists, these dark brown noodles are considered the best.

Udon and other white flour noodles

One of the most popular kinds of white flour noodle is udon. They are thick and white and have a wonderful chewy texture. They are eaten hot in soups with a variety of toppings, or cold with dipping sauce. Other tasty white flour noodles you might encounter include kishimen, which are chewy, flat and wide, almost like fettuccine. Somen are a snow white noodle as thin as angel hair pasta and almost always served cold in the summer. A slightly thicker version of somen is hiyamugi.

As with Italian pasta, I think fresh noodles taste the best. Throughout Japan, trained noodle masters sell hand-made soba and udon from their shops. However, since it's hard to find fresh soba and udon in the West, all the noodle recipes in this book call for dried noodles. But don't worry, high quality dried soba and udon are readily available and very tasty!

....

OILS

Rapeseed/canola oil

Polyunsaturates and, to a lesser extent, monounsaturates, have been shown to lower blood cholesterol levels and therefore help in reducing the risk of heart disease. It is better to eat foods rich in monounsaturates (olive oil and rapeseed oil) and polyunsaturates (sunflower oil and soya oil), than foods rich in saturates.

Rapeseed oil, which like olive oil contains mostly monounsaturated fat, is a good and cheaper alternative to olive oil. Rapeseed oil is one of the best vegetable oils to cook with, because it has among the highest concentrations of the good fats – polyunsaturated fat and monounsaturated fat – and the lowest of the bad kind of fat – saturated fat. And except in its hydrogenated form, it has absolutely none of the worst fat of all – trans fat.

Because rapeseed oil has little flavour, I find it allows the pure natural flavour of ingredients to shine through. For these reasons, I have called for it in all of my recipes, whenever a cooking oil is used. In Tokyo, my mother uses rapeseed oil for much of her frying and sautéing. She occasionally uses olive oil for Western dishes, which can handle the strong flavour of the oil, but olive oil is too overpowering for Japanese food. Look for *nonhydrogenated* rapeseed oil.

Sesame oil

Extracted from sesame seeds, sesame oil comes in two types: light and dark (also called toasted). The lighter oil has a softer flavour and colour than the dark version. Its potent flavour makes it appropriate to use as a garnish. My mother likes to drizzle dark sesame oil over hot-cooked foods because she finds the heat intensifies the oil's nutty flavour and aroma. Sesame oil can be used as cooking oil, but I seldom do since it burns too fast for my taste. Instead, I sprinkle it on stir-fried vegetables as soon as I turn off the heat and use it in my salad dressings (see page 170 for a recipe).

• • • • • • • • • • • • • •

Panko

Panko, Japanese breadcrumbs, is a modern ingredient, which makes a light, crunchy crust. (The term is a fusion of the French word for bread, *pain*, with *ko*, which means 'powder' in Japanese.) Unlike the breadcrumbs you are probably used to, panko have a texture that is more like flakes than crumbs.

Rice Vinegar

In addition to the fried, steamed and simmered categories of Japanese cooking, there is a fourth category: 'vinegared' dishes, typically served as starters or side dishes. The rice vinegar used in these dishes is made either from white rice or brown rice. Regular rice vinegar ranges in colour from light to golden yellow, while brown rice vinegar ranges from brown to black. Brown rice vinegar tastes milder than regular rice vinegar – yet rice vinegar overall has much less of a bite than pungent Western vinegars. Even when I'm making Western-style salads, I prefer to make my dressings with rice vinegar, since it's not as sour as white or red vinegar. If you have ever eaten sushi, you are already familiar with the taste of rice vinegar, since the sushi rice is gently tossed with a mixture of rice vinegar, sugar and salt.

Sake (rice wine)

Sake, which is made from fermented rice grains, not only makes a delightful alcoholic drink but also adds an indispensable touch to many Japanese dishes. Sake adds depth to simmered dishes, sauces and dressings and it reduces fish and meat odours.

Sake comes in numerous styles and, like wine, ranges enormously in quality, price and flavour, from dry to quite sweet. Use good-quality sake – the kind sold for drinking – when it comes to cooking. Just as most good Western cooks avoid 'cooking wine', steer clear from inexpensive so-called cooking sake because it contains added ingredients like sugar and salt that detract from, rather than enhance, the food. Since the alcohol in sake evaporates during cooking, you can still cook with it even if you avoid alcohol. Find it in an off-licence or the alcohol section of a supermarket.

. . . .

SEA VEGETABLES (SEAWEED)

Sea vegetables play an integral role in the Japanese diet. They are nutritious, tasty and extremely versatile. They are rich in iodine, folate, magnesium, iron, calcium, riboflavin and pantothenic acid. Sea vegetable-flavour stocks are found in cold salads, and they add a savoury crunch to rice and noodle dishes.

Kombu

Kombu, also known as konbu or kobu, is considered the king of seaweeds in Japan. A kind of kelp, it is thick, leafy and brownish green. Outside of Japan, kombu is primarily available dried, often in rectangles ranging in size from 2.5 x 13 cm (1 x 5 in) to 13 x 25 cm (5 x 10 in) for dashi. When steeped in water with dried bonito flakes, kombu makes the clear cooking stock dashi (see page 168), used as a basis for so many Japanese dishes. It's also enjoyed simmered (as an accompaniment to white rice) and dried as a snack.

Nori

Often called 'laver' outside of Japan, nori refers to the thin, flat sheets of dried seaweed that range in colour from pine green to purple black. If you've ever eaten sushi rolls, you've tasted nori. It's the crackly dark green substance that wraps around the vinegared rice (and eventually becomes soft and slightly chewy the longer it sits).

A popular Japanese snack that uses nori is *onigiri*, or rice balls. Every convenience store in Japan has a section devoted to these small vegetable- or fish-stuffed rice balls (or triangles) sealed with nori.

Nori used to make sushi is often toasted and comes labelled 'Sushi Nori'. Toasting enhances the flavour and crisp texture of the seaweed. Sushi nori usually comes in large 20-cm (8-in) squares with several sheets to a bag. Because nori loses its crispness as soon as it is exposed to air, remove only one sheet at a time for whatever you're making and keep the bag sealed at all times. To store, place the nori in an airtight container or zip-top bag.

Shredded nori makes a popular garnish for rice and noodle dishes. You can buy containers of commercially cut nori, or make your own, cutting a sheet of nori into a pile of 0.3 x 3-cm (¼ x 1-in) strips (or squares, as I sometimes do).

Seasoned nori sheets are also available. The crisp sheets are brushed with a sweet soy-based sauce and often sold in small rectangles with only a few sheets to each packet. Seasoned nori sheets wrapped around hot cooked rice are a popular Japanese breakfast treat and so easy to make. You simply take a small sheet of seasoned nori and quickly dip one side in some soy sauce. Then, wrap the seaweed around a mouthful of rice from your rice bowl. Alternatively, tear the seasoned nori into small bits and scatter them over your rice.

Wakame

Wakame is a common sea vegetable in Japan. Wakame is used in soups, salads and toppings for soba noodles everywhere. When you have miso soup at a Japanese restaurant, the chances are that it comes with a few ribbons of wakame. Inside Japan, you can buy fresh wakame – long green leaves. Outside of Japan, you can buy the dried version – dark green strands in a plastic bag.

• • • • • • • • • • • • • • •

Sesame Seeds (goma)

In Japanese home cooking, white and black sesame seeds add a fragrant, nutty accent to all kinds of dishes. I recommend buying whole sesame seeds untoasted. The seeds are used to garnish vegetable, tofu, seafood and meat dishes, as well as to flavour dipping sauces.

Grinding the seeds turns them into a flaky base used for

dressings and sauces. Most Japanese cooks grind their sesame seeds with a wooden mortar in a ribbed ceramic bowl called a *suribachi*. You can grind them in a food processor, or with a pestle and mortar. Or you can buy sesame seeds already ground.

Shichimi togarashi (seven-spice mix)
Shichimi togarashi adds a spicy, peppery flavour to foods. It is a distinctly Japanese blend of ground red pepper, roasted orange peel, white and black sesame seeds, Japanese pepper, seaweed and ginger. You could use ground cayenne, chilli peppers, if you cannot find *shichimi togarashi*, but it will add a kick of heat rather than the burst of heat and flavour you get from the combination of seven spices.

Shiso
Shiso is a herb in the mint family. Quite fragrant with a slightly bitter, mint-like flavour, shiso leaves are about 5 x 5 cm (2 x 2 in), heart-shaped with jagged edges. Shiso grows in green and reddish-purple colour varieties. Whole shiso leaves are commonly used in Japan as a garnish for sashimi and as an ingredient in tempura. Finely chopped leaves are used as a seasoning for tofu and other dishes and the dried chopped red leaves can be sprinkled on hot rice for flavouring. In early summer, pale pink shiso flowers on a short stem are used as a decorative and edible seasonal garnish. All shiso leaves used in my recipes are the green and fresh kind.

Shiso has a rich minty fragrance. Every time I open a packet of shiso, I bury my nose in the leaves and inhale deeply. I use whole leaves of it to wrap my rice balls and I often toss shredded shiso into my salads. In fact, I like shiso so much that I grow it in a planter at home.

Soy sauce (Shoyu)
Soy sauce, or *shoyu*, is a Japanese home-style cooking workhorse. This dark brown liquid, derived from soya beans, barley (or wheat), salt and water, has a distinctive savoury richness that gives Japanese cooking its signature flavour. In addition to seasoning soups, sauces, marinades and dressings, soy sauce serves as an indispensable condiment for dishes like sushi.

However, *soy sauce should be used with a delicate hand*. Many Westerners make the mistake of saturating their food with soy sauce, not realising that a little goes a very long way. When used properly and sparingly, soy sauce should bring out, not overwhelm, the innate flavour of an ingredient.

Because regular soy sauce contains high amounts of sodium, I feel it is one of the few non-healthy ingredients in the traditional Japanese larder if used to excess. (Some varieties of miso also suffer from the same high-sodium problem.)

However, there is a solution: use *reduced-sodium soy sauce*. To me, reduced-sodium soy sauce tastes just as good as, if not better than, regular soy sauce. Most supermarkets carry reduced-sodium soy sauce. All my recipes in this book call for reduced-sodium soy sauce.

When buying soy sauce, look for 'less salt', 'reduced salt', 'low salt' or 'reduced sodium' on the label. Be aware that the 'light (usukuchi)' variety can be misleading, and actually be higher in sodium content than regular soy sauce, and is only 'lighter' in liquid colour. Traditional Japanese cuisine chefs, especially in the Osaka and Kyoto area, prefer this type of soy sauce to achieve a clearer broth and to season ingredients, whether it's fish or vegetables, with flavours without darkening their natural colours. If you decide to use the light (usukuchi) soy sauce for these aesthetic reasons, I recommend that you further reduce the amount you use.

A high-quality wheat-free alternative to soy sauce that's popular among health food devotees and people with wheat allergies is *tamari*. It tastes similar to soy sauce and also comes in reduced-sodium varieties.

• • • • • • • • • • • • • • •

TOFU

Tofu is coagulated soya bean milk, made from soya beans and fashioned into blocks.

Most tofu is white with a hint of light yellow, like vanilla ice cream. Unlike in the USA, where tofu hasn't yet fully outlived its reputation as a hippie-inspired, tasteless health food, tofu is extremely popular in Japan. It's a sort of meat-and-potatoes ingredient for most Japanese home cooks and there are hundreds of delicious ways to prepare it.

Among tofu's many merits is its high-protein content. As a result, it makes a terrific substitute for all kinds of meats, poultry and seafood. When it's of good quality, it has a subtle, clean, lightly earthy taste.

Tofu is incredibly versatile. It can be added to starters, soups, main courses, dressings and desserts, as well as eaten on its own – hot or cold – with various garnishes. Tofu also delights the palate with its wide variety of textures, depending upon how it's prepared. Steaming, for example, turns tofu plump and juicy, while stir-frying turns it crispy, firm and golden. When stewed, tofu becomes tender and succulent and when whipped in a blender or food processor, it becomes creamy and thick, like soured cream (see page 171 for recipe).

Tofu is sold in various forms. The two basic kinds are known as 'silken' and 'cotton' (firm), and both may come in different degrees of firmness. Since the language used by different manufacturers to describe the several variations within those two general categories is not always consistent, here are some general directions to help you navigate through the tofu landscape.

Silken tofu

Silken tofu, or *kinugoshi* tofu, is extremely delicate, with a porcelain-like colour and a custard pudding-like texture both outside and inside. This lovely texture is achieved because silken tofu, unlike the firm types, are coagulated without being pressed to eliminate excess water.

For its external beauty and ever-so-subtle flavour, silken tofu is used in elegant soups, or chilled and eaten on its own with various garnishes.

Because silken tofu is so delicate, when my mother uses it she transfers the fragile tofu block directly from the container onto the palm of her left hand. She then uses her right hand to cut the tofu very carefully with a knife into bite-size or even smaller pieces. She then slides them with great care onto a plate or into water or broth that is gently simmering in a saucepan. All of this gentle handling is for the purpose of making sure that the tofu remains intact in little squares, which look so pretty floating, for instance, in a clear soup. If she were to cut the silken tofu on a chopping board, some pieces might break up when they are transferred from the chopping board to the saucepan or the plate.

Silken tofu is sold in airtight plastic containers with water, or in aseptic packaging without water. The waterless packaging means that it can keep indefinitely on the shelf. The water-packed variety has a shorter shelf life and should be used as soon as opened.

Firm tofu

Cotton (as it's known in Japan) or firm tofu, is less fragile than silken and, the 'firm' designation notwithstanding, it comes in textures generally labelled soft, medium firm, firm and extra firm. Generally speaking, the recipes in this book that call for cotton tofu use the firm texture, though that is more a matter of taste than necessity.

Cotton tofu is made by a different process from silken tofu, one that involves separating the curds from the whey of the soya milk and then compressing the curds. This is what makes the texture of cotton tofu so much firmer (even in its so-called soft versions). Cotton tofu has a slightly coarse surface and a much more substantial bite and texture than silken, which makes it suitable for stir-fries (see page 190 for a recipe) and for grilled and simmered dishes. It is almost always sold in water-filled cartons.

Yakidofu tofu

Yakidofu tofu is firm cotton tofu that has been grilled and has scorch marks on the surface. It's packed in water in a plastic container like the various kinds of cotton tofu, but tastes a tad smoky. It is used in sukiyaki dishes in Japan.

Because all tofu except the aseptically packed silken is quite perishable, be sure to use it within two days of purchase. Once opened, store it in the refrigerator submerged in cold water in a covered container.

• • • • • • • • • • • • • •

Yuzu (*Citrus junos*)

Yuzu is a popular citrus fruit. Its rind and juice are used to add a citrus aroma and sour taste to numerous Japanese dishes. Bottled yuzu juice is sold at Japanese speciality grocery stores. Fresh lime makes a good substitute.

Wasabi

Wasabi is a popular Japanese condiment that suffuses the palate with a mixture of spice and heat. Unlike the horseradish plant, which grows in soil, wasabi grows in cold, shallow streams high in the mountains of Japan. The rhizome portion of the wasabi plant, which is the edible part, is about 2.5 cm (1 in) in diameter and ranges from 8 to 15 cm (3 to 6 in) long. Wasabi is expensive to harvest and cultivate, which is why most shops sell a cheap substitute under the wasabi name. If you've ever eaten sushi or sashimi at a modestly priced Japanese restaurant, chances are you've been served a small cone of light green paste fabricated primarily from mustard and/or horseradish powder and green food colouring. It's acrid, fiery and flavourless and bears little resemblance to freshly grated wasabi.

Beyond its use in sushi and sashimi, wasabi often accompanies cold soba noodles, chilled tofu and various fish and grilled chicken dishes.

TOKYO KITCHEN UTENSILS – USEFUL TO KNOW/HAVE

Drop-lid (*otoshi buta*)

A drop-lid, or *otoshi buta*, is a low-tech device for simmering. Simmering happens a lot in my mother's Tokyo kitchen, with vegetables, meat and fish. A Japanese drop-lid is flat and made of wood and, instead of resting on top of the pot like a conventional lid, it sits directly on the ingredients inside. By staying so close to the food, it re-channels the broth through all the ingredients, maximising the natural flavours of the food. A drop-lid should be a bit smaller than the diameter of the pot interior.

Otoshi-buta drop-lids are hard to find in shops outside of Japan, but look for one at a shop that carries Japanese cooking tools. Alternatively, you can fashion a substitute with kitchen foil. Cut a double layer of foil in a circle a bit smaller than the interior of your pot or pan and lay it on top of the food you're simmering. When a pot is too small for my drop-lid, I use this method. It works very well.

Non-stick rice paddle (*shamoji*)

To fluff up cooked rice without squashing the grains, the Japanese have developed a non-stick rice paddle with small bumps on the surfaces. You can find it at any store that stocks Japanese cookware. An electronic rice cooker often comes with its own rice paddle and a measuring cup.

Wooden sushi tub (*hangiri sushi oke*)

This is a tub designed to absorb extra moisture from the rice and vinegar mixture.

RESOURCES

A number of supermarkets carry Japanese foods and ingredients. They may be found in the 'Oriental Foods' section and scattered elsewhere in the shop. For less-common Japanese ingredients, your best source is a Japanese speciality grocery store, or online stores. Gourmet and health food stores stock select Japanese items as well. For fresh vegetables and fruits, don't forget to visit your local farmers' and organic markets.

Here are some (by no means all) resources for finding basic staples, Japanese ingredients and Japan-style cookware and tableware.

UK

Farmers' Markets

Certified Farmers' Markets
http://www.farmersmarkets.net/

London Farmers' Markets
www.lfm.org.uk

Japanese Speciality Stores and Online Shopping

Japan Centre Food Shop
www.japancentre.com
212 Piccadilly, London W1J 9HG
Tel: 020-7434-4218
One of the biggest Japanese markets in the UK, with over 1,000 items direct from Japan, including rice, seaweeds, sauces, sake, edamame, sake, dashi, miso and green teas.

Japanese Kitchen
www.japanesekitchen.co.uk
9 Lower Richmond Road, Putney, London SW15 1EJ
Tel: 020-8788-9014
A wide selection of Japanese short-grain rice, soy sauce, mirin, vinegar, green teas, panko, sesame seeds and sea vegetables.

Mount Fuji International
www.mountfuji.co.uk
Nr Shrewsbury SY4 1AS
Japanese food ingredients and seasonings, green teas, barley tea, tableware and rice cookers.
Tel: 01743-741169

Arigato
48–50 Brewer Street, London W1F 9TG
Tel: 020-7287-1722
This Japanese supermarket in Soho's 'Little Tokyo' carries the essentials, from nori, soy sauce and tofu to Japanese sake and beer.

Atari-Ya Food
Acton:
7 Station Parade, Noel Road, London W3 0DS
Tel: 020-8896-1552
Finchley:
595 High Road, North Finchley, London N12 0DY
Tel: 020-8446-6669

Cardiff Korean & Japanese Foods
116 Woodville Road, Cathays, Cardiff CF24 4EE
Tel: 029-2022-3225

Fuji Foods
167 Priory Road, London N8 8NB
Tel: 020-8347-9177

Fuji Food Store Cambridge
The Shopping Forum 18–22 Jesus Lane, Cambridge, Cambridgeshire CB5 8QB
Tel: 01223-308008

J-mart
Oriental City, 399 Edgware Road, London NW9 0JJ
Tel: 020-8205-3988

The Japanese Shop
http://www.thejapaneseshop.co.uk/
Tableware, gifts and bento boxes.

Minamoto Kitchoan
http://www.kitchoan.com/
44 Piccadilly, London W1J ODS
Tel: 020-7437-3135
Top-quality traditional Japanese sweets.

Muji
http://www.mujionline.co.uk/home/Stores.asp (store locations)
http://www.mujionline.co.uk/online/online.asp?V=1&Sec=4 (E-commerce)
Contemporary Japanese kitchenware.

Natural Natural
Ealing Common:
20 Station Parade, Uxbridge Rd, London W5 3LD
Tel: 020-8992-0770
Finchley Road:
1 Goldhurst Terrace, London NW6 3HX
Tel: 020-7624-5734

Oki-Nami Japanese Shop
www.okinami.com
12 York Place, Brighton, East Sussex BN1 4GU
Tel: 01273-677702

Oriental City Supermarket
399 Edgware Road, London NW9 0JJ
Tel: 020-8200-0009

Rice Wine
82 Brewer Street, London W1F 9UA
Tel: 020-7439-3705
Japanese food ingredients and seasonings, green teas, tableware
and rice cookers.

Saki Delicatessen & Food Boutique
http://www.saki-food.com
4 West Smithfield, London EC1A 9JX
Tel: 020-7489-7033

Gourmet and Speciality Stores

Clearspring
www.clearspring.co.uk
http://www.goodnessdirect.co.uk (Ecommerce)
Manufacturer of miso, soba, tofu, daikon, nori, kombu, mirin and other products.

Harrod's
www.harrods.com
87 Brompton Road London SW1X 7XL
Gourmet food halls, including sushi bar.

Harrods 102
102 Brompton Road, London SW3 1JJ
Tel: 020-7730-1234
A luxury late-opening convenient store with healthy choices.

Harvey Nichols
109–125 Knightsbridge, London SW1X 7RJ
Tel: 020-7235-5000

Marks & Spencer
http://www.marksandspencer.com/
Gourmet food halls.

Partridges
www.partridges.co.uk
2–5 Duke of York Square, London SW3 4LY
Tel: 020-7730-0651

Panzers Delicatessen
http://www.panzers.co.uk
13–19 Circus Road, St John's Wood, London NW8 6PB
Tel: 020-7722-8596
Global gourmet deli, including Japanese items.

Planet Organic
25 Effie Road, Fulham, London SW6 1EL
Tel: 020-7731-7222
42 Westbourne Grove, London W2 5SH
Tel: 020-7727-2227
22 Torrington Place, London WC1 7JE
Tel: 020-7436-1929

Selfridges & Co.
http://www.selfridges.com/
Gourmet food halls, including Yo! Sushi.

The Spice Shop
www.thespiceshoponline.com/acatalog/index.html
1 Blenheim Crescent, London W11 2EE
Tel: 020-7221-4448
Japanese Products section has miso, sesame seeds, sea
vegetables, mirin, shichimi togarashi, soba, udon, soy sauce,
toasted sesame oil and wasabi.

Whole Foods Market + Fresh & Wild
http://wholefoodsmarket.com/stores/list_UK.html
The world's largest organic and natural retailer.

Camden Town:
49 Parkway, London NW1 7PN
Tel: 020-7428-7575

Clapham Junction:
305–311 Lavender Hill, London SW11 1LN
Tel: 020-7585-1488

Clifton, Bristol:
85 Queen's Road, Bristol BS8 1QS
Tel: 0117-910-5930

Kensington:
Kensington High Street, London
(opening 2007)

Notting Hill:
208–212 Westbourne Grove, London W11 2RH
Tel: 020-7229-1063

Soho:
69–75 Brewer Street, London W1F 9US
Tel: 020-7434-3179

Stoke Newington:
32–40 Stoke Newington Church Street, London N16 0LU
Tel: 020-7254-2332

Supermarkets

Waitrose
www.waitrosedeliver.com
Stocks Japanese items such as nori sea vegetables, soy sauce, mirin, sake, wasabi, rice vinegar, ginger, Asian pear, green tea, persimmon, shiitake mushroom and sweet potatoes.

Sainsbury
www.sainsburys.co.uk
Has Japanese items including soy sauce, rice vinegar, tofu, miso, wasabi and Fuji apples.

Tesco
www.tesco.com
Carries sushi rice, tofu, udon, daikon, shiitake mushrooms, Fuji apples, rice vinegar, soy sauce and sake.

ASDA
http://www.asda.co.uk

Marks and Spencer
http://www.marksandspencer.com

Budgens
http://www.budgens.co.uk/

Morrisons
http://www.morrisons.co.uk/

Japanese Takeaways

itsu
http://www.itsu.co.uk/shops/

Yo! Sushi
http://www.yosushi.com/

wasabi sushi and bento
http://www.wasabi.uk.com/

Online Gateways

www.amazon.co.uk
Home & Garden section stocks rice cookers, woks and Oriental tableware.

http://froogle.google.co.uk/
Japanese ingredients, tableware and cookware.

http://shopping.yahoo.co.uk
Home & Garden section leads you to the Japanese ingredients,
cooking tools and Oriental tableware.

AUSTRALIA

Japanese Grocery

Anegawa
Shop 10, 7–17 Waters Road, Neutral Bay NSW 20
Tel: 02-9904-4177
16A Deepwater Road, Castle Cove NSW 20
Tel: 02-9417-5452

Ichibankan
36 Muse Walk, The Rocks, 2000
Tel: 02-9247-2667

JUSCO Supermarket
Level 6, Westfield Shoppingtown, Chatswood
Tel: 02-9419-8933

Maruya
Basement 283–285 Clarence Street, Sydney, NSW 2000
Tel: 02-9267-0888

My Mart
Level 2, 10–14 Bulletin Place, Sydney 2000 NSW
Tel: 02-9251-8732

Tokyo Mart
Located in Northbridge Plaza
79–113 Sailors Bay Road, Northbridge NSW 262
Tel: 02-9958-6860
A comprehensive Japanese grocery.

Usagi-ya
1/314 Oxford Street, Bondi Junction NSW 2
Tel: 02-9369-3121

Ume-ya
Shop 3, Crows Nest Plaza
103–111 Willoughby Rd, Crows Nest, NSW 2065

Gourmet and Speciality Stores

David Jones
Foodhall, Market Street, Sydney
www.davidjones.com.au

Harris Farm Markets
http://www.harrisfarm.com.au

macro wholefoods market
http://www.macrowholefoods.com.au

The Sydney Fish market
Bank Street Pyrmont, NSW 2009
Tel: 02-9004-1100
www.sydneyfishmarket.com.au

Paddy's Markets
www.paddysmarkets.com.au

The Sydney Fresh Food Market
Building D at Sydney Markets
Parramatta Road, Flemington

The Essential Ingredient
www.theessentialingredient.com.au/locations.html

PK Superstores
303 Penshurst Street
Willoughby NSW
Tel: 02-9882-1822

Prahran Market
163 Commercial Road, South Yarra 3141 Victoria
http://www.prahranmarket.com.au/traderList.html

Supermarkets

Woolworths
www.woolworths.com.au/

Coles Supermarkets
http://www.coles.com.au/

Takeaways

Simmone Logue
www.simmonelogue.com

Kabocha
Shop 6, 8 Waters Road, Neutral Bay, NSW 2089
Tel: 02-9953-0379

Makers

SunRice
www.sunrice.com.au/
Rice growers in Australia, make Japanese short-grain
Koshihikari sushi rice and 90-second microwaveable short-grain
brown rice.

Sun Masamune
http://www.sun-masamune.com.au/home.htm
Australian sake manufacturer.

NEW ZEALAND

Japan Mart
75 Anzac Ave, Auckland, Central Auckland
Tel: 0-9-377-2226

The Mediterranean Markets
www.mediterranean.co.nz
53 Robins Road, The Junction, Queenstown
50 Reece Crescent, Wanaka
122 Town Centre, Te Anau

Auckland Fish Market
http://www.afm.co.nz/
Corner of Daldy and Madden Streets
Freemans Bay, Auckland
Tel: 0-9-379-1490

New World
www.newworld.co.nz/StoreLocations/Default.aspx

Woolworths
https://www.woolworths.co.nz

Foodtown Supermarkets
www.foodtown.co.nz

Resources on Health, Diet and Nutrition:

- UK Food Standards Agency 'Eatwell' website
  Information on healthy diet and obesity, plus body mass
  index (BMI) calculator: http://www.eatwell.gov.uk

- British Dietetic Association:
  http://www.bda.uk.com/
  http://www.bdaweightwise.com/bda/

- UK Food Standards Agency Balance of Good Health:
  http://www.food.gov.uk/multimedia/pdfs/bghbooklet.pdf

- Fish Safety and Sustainability
  http://www.fishonline.org/
  http://www.scottishsalmon.co.uk/
  http://www.puresalmon.org/seafood.html
  http://www.mcsuk.org/
  http://www.seafoodchoices.com/smartchoices.php
  http://www.oceansalive.org/eat.cfm?subnav=bestandworst
  http://www.seafoodwatch.org
  http://www.fishonline.org/information/MCSPocket_Good_Fis
  h_Guide.pdf

Author Website:

Visit us at www.thejapandiet.com for more resources and web
links on health, diet and nutrition.

SOURCE NOTES

Quotations from experts not cited below are from interviews with the authors.

Information and quotations from the Food Standards Agency, the Department of Health, the British Dietetic Association, the World Health Organization, Heart UK, Cancer Research UK, the International Obesity Task Force, the American Dietetic Association, the American Institute for Cancer Research and the U.S. National Institutes of Health not cited below are from those organisations' websites, consulted in the summer and autumn of 2006.

Day 1: Step Into a Dieter's Dream
'Learn all the rules, then forget them': Kakuzo Okakura, *The Book of Tea* (Boston: Shambhala, 2001), p. xii.
'If eaten in the balance that the Japanese apply': Registered Dietitian Jane Kirby, who runs the Vermont Cooking School & Farm, said this in an author interview. She also made this point in her book, Jane Kirby and American Dietetic Association, *Dieting for Dummies* (New York: Wiley Publishing, 2004), p. 178.

DAY 2: Come with Me to Tokyo
Japanese government considers 1980 as the point of nutritional balance: 'What is Food Education?' Japanese Ministry of Agriculture, Forestry and Fisheries: www.maff.go.jp/english_p/shokuiku.pdf

DAY 3: Understand Why Fad Diets Aren't Working
'When you look at the number of people': Valerie Elliott, 'Junk food has claimed a generation', *The Times*, 24 October 2005.
30,000 premature deaths from obesity, obesity tripled since 1980: *Tackling Obesity in England: Report by the Comptroller and Auditor General*, 8 February 2001.
www.nao.gov.uk/publications/nao_reports/00-01/0001220es.pdf

'In the last decade British children': John Carvel, 'Child obesity has doubled in a decade', *The Guardian,* 22 April 2006.

U.S. Surgeon General on 'terror' and magnitude of obesity: Katrina A. Jackson, 'Surgeon General says Americans must address obesity', *Associated Press,* 1 March 2006.

'It is just staggering': Daniel DeNoon, 'Obesity epidemic balloons to new girth', *WebMD Medical News,* 4 April 2006.

'We are eating too much saturated fat': Madeleine Brindley, 'Cut gimmicks and sell healthy food as main choice', *The Western Mail,* 4 May 2006.

Schwartz–Woloshin analysis: Lindsey Tanner, 'Medical journal puts itself and its competitors under the microscope', *Associated Press,* 8 June 2002.

'The reality is we don't know': Kitta MacPherson, 'Researchers nibble away at the problem of obesity', *The Star-Ledger* (Newark, NJ), 9 April 2003.

'It's amazing how few good studies', Bonnie Leibman and David Schardt, 'The Sure-Fire…Diet', *Nutrition Action Healthletter,* 1 January 2004.

'Nothing is ever as straightforward': Lois Rogers, 'Kill or cure?' *The Sunday Times,* 1 January 2006.

DAY 4: Open the Holy Grail of Diets

'Patients need to understand': Dr John J. Whyte, Dr Robert N. Marting, 'How to guide patients away from fad diets and toward healthy eating', *Patient Care,* 1 May 2005.

'People who succeed at maintaining a dramatic weight loss': Carla K. Johnson, 'New study refutes claims by promoters of Atkins, Zone diets', *Associated Press-CanWest News Service, Vancouver Sun,* 9 January 2006.

'What the scientific evidence says' chart: adapted from 'Diet, Nutrition and the Prevention of Chronic Diseases', WHO Technical Report Series 916, Report of a Joint WHO/FAO Expert Consultation, Geneva, 28 January–1 February 2002; report published 23 April 2003, Chapter 5, 'Population nutrient intake goals for preventing diet-related chronic diseases'; Table 7, 'Summary of strength of evidence on factors that might promote or protect against weight gain and obesity' and associated notes.

'A calorie is a calorie is a calorie': 'Profile: Low-carb diet food expands to more and more products', NBC News, *Today,* 23 June 2004.

DAY 6: How the Japanese Diet Compares with the UK Diet

Figures on daily calorie supply per person are from the United Nations FAO Balance Sheets posted on the Food and Agricultural Organization's website: http://faostat.fao.org/?alias=faostatclassic

DAY 7: Open Your Mind to the Japan Diet Attitude

Dictionary definitions of 'diet': Webster's Revised Unabridged Dictionary 1913, accessed online.

'The whole concept of a diet': Mary Papadakis, Rhiannon Hoyle, 'Fighting the Flab', *Sunday Mail*, 18 July 2004.

'Pick one or two changes': Michelle Meadows, 'Healthier Eating', *FDA Consumer* magazine May–June 2005, http://www.fda.gov/fdac/ features /2005/305_eat.html

'The key is moderation': Dr John J. Whyte, Dr Robert N. Marting, 'How to guide patients away from fad diets and toward healthy eating', *Patient Care,* 1 May 2005.

DAY 9: Step into a Beautiful World – Right Around the Corner

'They have rites and customs so different': Paul Varley and Kumakura Isao, *Tea in Japan: Essays on the History of Chanoyu* (Honolulu: University of Hawaii Press, 1989), p. 103.

'The most exciting restaurant city in the world': Nancy Kruse, 'The Kruse Report, London chains lead the way', *Nation's Restaurant News*, 5 December 2005.

'Japanese cuisine could soon be as common': Simon Beckett, 'Soy successful', *The Independent on Sunday,* 5 June 2005.

Tesco selling more sushi than cheese sandwiches: Michael Fitzpatrick, 'Japanese cool cuisine set to conquer the world', *Just-Food,* 26 October 2005.

'We're talking big': Alex Renton, 'How sushi ate the world', *The Observer,* 26 February 2006.

Ms. Lowden on sushi: Molly Watson, 'Forget soggy sarnies at your desk', *The Western Mail,* 21 August 2006.

DAY 10: See the Beauty of Mindful Eating

'When you eat, eat slowly': Lydia Forbes, 'On the Business of Life', *Forbes Global,* 25 July 2005.

'Eating fast may lead to obesity': Sally Squires, 'Take your time at the plate', *Times Union* (Albany, NY), 28 December 2005.

'Eating slowly may provide more time': 'Why eating slowly may help you slim', *Daily Mail,* 29 June 2000.

'Eat too quickly': Peter Jaret, 'Taming your primal appetite', *Natural Health,* 1 July 2004.

'You have to give your body time to understand': Fran Henry, 'Slow eating can improve your health', *Times-Picayune* (New Orleans, Louisiana), 15 July 2005.

DAY 11: Liberate Your Dishes and Humanise Your Portions

'Everything is so big here': Hannah Karp and Ginny Parker Woods, 'Big in Vegas: Sumo Wrestling', *The Wall Street Journal*, 7 October 2005.

'Is that the size for the American people': Jenny Hontz, 'The One U.S. City Outsize Enough for Sumo', *The New York Times*, 10 October 2005.

'Studies show that people tend to passively overeat': Peter Jaret, 'Taming your primal appetite', *Natural Health*, 1 July 2004.

'By American standards, the courses Japanese eat': Peggy Orenstein, 'Japanese Lessons', *Health* magazine, April 2003.

'They come alive in amazing transfiguration': Yoshio Tsuchiya, *A Feast for the Eyes: The Japanese Art of Food Arrangement* (New York: Kodansha, 1985), p. 35.

'Design a pattern or image', 'has a beauty of its own': ibid., p. 36.

DAY 12: Colour Your Life with Fruit and Vegetables

Benefits of fruits and vegetables: Willett, *Eat, Drink, and be Healthy*, page 132.

'One way of getting a good variety': Annie Pierce Rusunen, 'Power Foods: Plant Foods Help Ward Off Diseases', *The Columbian* (Vancouver, Washington), 9 April 2002.

'Fruits and vegetables really are key players': Shirley Wang and Betsy McKay, 'More Reasons to Eat Your Veggies', *The Wall Street Journal*, 25 July 2006.

'Surprisingly, foods with a high water content': Barbara Rolls and Robert Barnett, *The Volumetrics Weight-Control Plan* (New York: Quill, 2000).

'Many people who know a little about phytochemicals': American Institute of Cancer Research press release, 'A Closer Look at Phytochemicals', 23 June 2006.

'It is likely, that the combination of nutrients': Lyn M. Steffen, 'Eat your fruit and vegetables', *The Lancet*, 28 January 2006.

'Because lengthy cooking can damage': Walter Willett and Molly Katzen, *Eat, Drink and Weigh Less* (New York: Hyperion, 2006), p. 20.

Wall Street Journal list of fruits and vegetables: Shirley Wang and Betsy McKay, 'More Reasons To Eat Your Veggies', *The Wall Street Journal*, 25 July 2006.

DAY 13: Have a Japan-Style Vegetable Moment

'A nutritional All–Star': Center for Science in the Public Interest, *Nutrition Action Health Letter*, 'Ten Super Foods for Better Health', 2006.

Quotes and news on sweet potato in UK: 'How the sweet potato is growing on us', *Daily Mail*, 16 May 2006.

Seaweed in the UK: Charles Campion, 'Seaweed is making a ripple', *The Evening Standard*, 24 May 2006.

The FSA has advised against eating one form of seaweed, called hijiki, due to its high levels of inorganic arsenic, a possible carcinogen. 'If you have eaten hijiki occasionally,' the FSA added in a 2004 statement, 'it is unlikely that you will have raised your risk significantly of getting cancer.' Hijiki has not been banned, and is available in some Japanese markets.

DAY 14: Swim in the Good Fats – with Fish

'It is clear that we cannot swallow all the hype': Joe Schwarcz, 'Omega-3 study nets a fishy controversy', *Montreal Gazette,* 8 July 2006.

Farmed salmon criticised: for example, see the article published by David Carpenter and colleagues, 'Global Assessment of Organic Contaminants in Farmed Salmon', *Science,* 9 January 2004.

'Are likely to be at least 100-fold greater': Sally Squires, 'Good Fish, Bad Fish', *The Washington Post,* 8 August 2006.

DAY 15: Try Some Soya

Figures on daily protein supply per person are from the FAO Balance Sheets posted on the Food and Agricultural Organization's website: http://faostat.fao.org/?alias=faostatclassic

The edamame section is reprinted with permission from the American Institute for Cancer Research.

Opinions of Agency for Healthcare Research and Quality, Dr Marion Nestle on soya: James Nestor, 'Too Much of a Good Thing?' *San Francisco Chronicle,* 13 August 2006.

Soya associated with small reduction in breast cancer risk: American Institute of Cancer Research press release, 'New Soy-Breast Cancer Study Finds Small but Significant Protective Effect', 4 April 2006. For full details, see: http://www.aicr.org/site/News2?abbr=pr_&page=NewsArticle&id=9679

American Heart Association on soya: 'Soy protein shows little effect on "bad" cholesterol', AHA scientific statement, American Heart Association scientific statement: 17 January, 2006. http://www.americanheart.org/presenter. jhtml?identifier=3037031

For a very detailed report on the possible health and safety implications of phytoestrogens in the diet, see:

'Phytoestrogens and Health', report by Food Standards Agency Committee on Toxicity of Chemicals in Food, published 1 May 2003, available at: http://www.food.gov.uk/multimedia/pdfs/ phytoreport0503

DAY 16: Unleash the Power of Rice and Wholegrains

'A darkly gleaming lidded lacquer bowl': Amanda Mayer Stinchecum, 'Japanese Rice in Its Many Guises', *The New York Times,* 25 March 1990.

Dr Walter Willett on using white rice sparingly: see 'The New Healthy

Eating Pyramid', *Eat, Drink and Be Healthy,* p. 13.

Study of 1,354 Japanese female farmers: 'Metabolic risk factors in Japanese women consuming traditional diet examined', *Diabetes Week,* 10 July 2006.

Japanese researchers arguing that short-grain white rice should *not* be classified as high GI: Tatsuhiro Matsuo, Yasuhiro Mizushima, Maki Komuro, Akiko Sugeta and Masashige Suzuki; 'Estimation of glycemic and insulinemic responses to short-grain rice (Japonica) and a short-grain rice-mixed meal in healthy young subjects', *Asia Pacific Journal of Clinical Nutrition,* September 1999, p. 190.

Also, the University of Sydney GI database (www.glycemicindex.com) reports a very wide range of GI scores for different tests of different types of white rice: from a low GI of 38 for 'Converted rice, white, boiled 20–30 min, Uncle Ben's® brand', to a high GI of 139 for 'White rice, boiled, low-amylose (Turkey)'.

The FSA has this advice on storing and reheating rice: 'There are a few things to remember when you are storing and reheating cooked rice and grains. This is because the spores of some food poisoning bugs can survive cooking. If cooked rice or grains are left standing at room temperature, the spores can germinate. The bacteria multiply and produce toxins that can cause vomiting and diarrhoea. Reheating food won't get rid of the toxins. Therefore, it's best to serve rice and grains when they've just been cooked. If this isn't possible, cool them within an hour after cooking and keep them refrigerated until reheating or using in a cold dish. You should throw away any rice and grains that have been left at room temperature overnight. Don't keep cooked rice and grains for longer than two days and don't reheat them more than once. Check the 'use by' date and storage instructions on the label for any cold rice or grain salads that you buy.'

'Let simple seem like much': Shizuo Tsuji, *Japanese Cooking: A Simple* Art (Tokyo: Kodansha International, 1980), p. 16.

'Stay simple!': ibid., p. 14.

Naomichi Ishige quotes: Naomichi Ishige, *The History and Culture of Japanese Food* (London: Kegan Paul, 2001), p. 225.

'A hand moves, and the fire's whirling': Stephen Mitchell, ed., *The Enlightened Heart: An Anthology of Sacred Poetry* (New York: HarperPerennial, 1989), p. 36. Passage translated by Stephen Mitchell.

'It is a cuisine – it is difficult to call it cooking': Jeremy Ferguson, 'Tastes of Japan', *The Globe and Mail* (Toronto), 15 August 1990.

DAY 18: Lighten Up Your Beverages

Clinton's being 'stuffed' with food as a child, food details and weight struggles: Sharon Cotliar, 'Loss Leader', *People Magazine,* 14 November 2005; Sanjay Gupta and Elizabeth Cohen, 'Bill Clinton and Weight', *CNN: House Call with Dr Sanjay Gupta,* 6 August 2005; Lawrence K. Altman,

'Clinton joins fight against child obesity', *The New York Times*, 4 May 2005. Also, see Bill Clinton, *My Life* (New York : Knopf, 2004), pages 14 and 15 Clinton and pizza in Oval Office: 'Pizza de Resistance', *The Sunday Times*, 25 September 1994. Clinton's food consumption during one day (eggs, sausage, scrapple, cheesecake, pizza, frozen yogurt, etc.): Frank J. Murray, 'Bubba returns for pizza, bowling in Hot Springs', *The Washington Times*, 29 December 1993. Clinton ate up to seven meals in one day: Clinton aide Paul Begala quoted in Susan Schindehette, Sharon Cotliar, Diane Herbst, Marianne V. Stochmal, Macon Morehouse, Linda Kramer, 'Midlife Crisis', *People Magazine*, 20 September 2004. Additional details of Clinton weight and heart surgery: Sam Dolnick, 'Clinton has successful quadruple bypass', Associated Press, 6 September 2004. 'This one policy can add years and years': Tom Baldwin, 'Coca-Cola excludes itself from American education', *The Times*, 4 May 2006.

'Disordered lifestyle', 'they sit in front of the telly': Camillo Fracassini, 'Proved: TV leads to junk food diet', *The Sunday Times*, 9 April 2006.

'Tea tempers the spirit': Richard R. Powell, *Wabi Sabi Simple* (Avon MA: Adams Media, 2005), p. 81.

Green and black tea sales in the UK, 2000 to 2005: Leo Lewis, 'The man who plans to turn the world green', *The Times*, 29 April 2006, citing Euromonitor data.

'The consumption of six to 10 cups of tea per day': John Fauber, 'Debate rages over benefits, risks of tea, coffee', *Charleston Gazette* (Virginia), 3 July 2006.

Japanese green tea study of over 40,000 adults: Lindsey Tanner, 'Green Tea: Mixed Review As Health Aid', Associated Press, 12 September 2006.

DAY 20: Jumpstart with Breakfast

'Eating breakfast is a characteristic common': Holly Wyatt, Gary Grunwald, Cecilia Mosca, Mary Klem, James Hill, Rena Wing; 'Long-term weight loss and breakfast in subjects in the National Weight Control Registry', *Obesity Research*, 2 February 2002. Note: this study was funded in part by the General Mills breakfast cereal company.

DAY 21: Integrate Your Exercise

'I regret preaching the doctrine of aerobics', 'You don't have to push yourself': Tara Parker-Pope, 'Why Your New Year's Resolution to Get Healthier May Be Pretty Easy to Keep', *The Wall Street Journal*, 3 January 2006.

Dr Till comments: Lucy Atkins, 'Gym'll fix it?' *Daily Telegraph*, 11 March 2006.

'People don't fail in losing weight': Susan Stevens, 'New year, new diet', *Chicago Daily Herald*, 3 January 2005.

Study of 73,000 adults in Japan: 'Walking and Sports Linked with Heart Health Benefits in Japan, Too', American College of Cardiology news release, 1 November 2005.

'The everyday lives of most people': Nanci Hellmich, 'Our big gain will be our loss': *USA Today,* 19 July 2004.

'The activity levels of people in the 1950s', 'It is no good squeezing all this extra activity': Peta Bee, 'Walking the dog will work for owners', *The Times,* 29 April 2006.

'Walking is an accessible, inexpensive': 'Exercise cuts stroke risk in women', *Reuters,* 13 June 2000.

Estimates of calorie expenditures from physical activities are from American Institute of Cancer Research report, 'A Closer Look at Energy Balance', available online at:

http://www.aicr.org/site/PageServer?pagename=pub_eb

DAY 30: The Days of Magical Eating . . . and an Eternal Love Affair with Food

'When with the first month comes the spring': *The Manyoshu: the Nippon Gakujutsu Shinkokai Translation of One Thousand Poems* (New York: Columbia University Press, 1965), p. 241.

'Many curious and beautiful things have vanished': Lafcadio Hearn, *Gleanings in Buddha Fields* (Boston: Houghton Mifflin, 1897), p. 52.

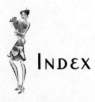

INDEX

Abdel-Hady, Tarik 75
Alaska Salmon 155–6
Andoh, Elizabeth 218
ASDA 'Good for You' range 151
Asparagus Salad with White Sesame
    Dressing 184
Atkins Diet 18
Aubergine & Green Peppers with
    Red Miso Dressing 193–4

Balance of Good Health' eating plan
    20
Bananas on Toasted Multi-grain
    Bread 214
Barnett, Robert 68
BDA (British Dietetic Association) 3,
    4, 17, 20, 22
    health benefits of wholegrains
        93
    meaning of BMI ranges 41
    waist measurements 41–2
Beckett, Simon 46
Beef, Sweet Potato and Onion
    Casserole – one pot dish 206–7
Beetroot Leaves Salad with Lemon
    Dressing 187
Bento Box 62–3
beverages 105–12
    brewing Japanese teas 111–12
    green tea 108–9
    healthy choices 108–10
    Japanese teas 219–21
    sweetened fizzy drinks 105–7
BMI (body mass index) 10, 15
    calculation 40

meaning of different levels 41
Body and Soul Warming Soba
    Buckwheat Noodles with
    Sardine & Spinach 209–10
bonito (fish) flakes (katsuo-bushi,
    hana-katsuo or kezuribushi)
    217
breakfast 119–22
    benefits of 121
    importance for weight control
        121–2
    Japanised-Western 8–9
    quick healthy options 122
    sample meals based on recipes
        161–2
breast cancer rates in Japan 88
breast cancer risk, and soya 88–9
brown rice 91–8
    Brown Rice (recipe) 156
    health benefits 92–3
    types of Japanese rice 93–6
    variety of uses 91–2
    ways to eat more 96–7
Buckley, Dr John 126

Caballero, Dr Benjamin 89, 95
calorie density of foods 68
calories
    and weight loss 23
    comparison of UK and Japanese
        diets 29–31
cancer incidence, Japan 28, 88
carbohydrates, confusion about 18
cardiovascular disease 15
Carmona, Richard 15

Cauliflower–Napa Cabbage 'East-Meets-West' Soup 180
chicken recipes
    Chicken & Eggs (Parent & Child) over Fluffy Rice 205–6
    Japanese Country Style Simmered Chicken, Broccoli & Carrot 204–5
Chilled Cucumber Salad 185
Clinton, Bill 105–6
Co-op 'Healthy Living' range 151
Collins, Karen 68, 89
Colquhoun, Dr David 7
cooking Japan-style
    cooking methods 101–4
    food philosophy 99–101
    simmering 102
    steaming 102–4
    vinegared dishes 102
Cool Summer Soba Buckwheat Noodle Salad 208–9
coronary heart disease
    effects of the Japanese diet 78–9
    rates in Japan 78–9
Corrigan, Richard 76
cotton tofu 230
crash diets see fad diets
Creamy Tofu Sauce 171

daikon (large white radish) 217
Dansinger, Dr Michael 21
Dashi – Japanese Fish Cooking Stock 168–9
dessert 157
diabetes 15
diet, definitions 32
'Dietary Approaches to Stop Hypertension' (DASH) 20, 73
dieting
    criticism of 17
    lack of proper research on 17–19
    see also fad diets
Dietz, Dr William 12–13
dinner
    Japan-style 9
    quick and easy Japan-style menu 154–8
    sample meals based on recipes 163–4

dressings
    Sesame Oil Salad Dressing 170
    Toasted & Ground White Sesame Seeds 171
    Traditional Japanese Vinaigrette 170
    White Sesame Seed Dressing 172
drop-lid (otoshi buta) 232

eating speed
    and overeating 53–4
    and weight gain 53–4
    mindful eating 50–3
Eckel, Dr Robert 17
edamame (fresh green soya beans) 87, 218
    Edamame Mesclun Salad 186
    Rice with Edamame Soya Beans 173
eggs, Chicken & Eggs (Parent & Child) over Fluffy Rice 205–6
energy density of foods 68
Escoffier, Auguste 100
exercise 123–30
    and weight loss 125
    benefits of walking 127
    health benefits 126–6
    integrative exercise 124–6, 127–30
    levels in everyday life 124–6
    low-intensity 123
    track your progress 129–30
    ways to fit more into your life 127–30

fad diets 3
    attitude 32, 33
    why they don't work 14, 15–19
farmers' markets 115–16
fats in the diet 23
    bad 80
    good 81
    monounsaturated 81
    non-hydrogenated 81
    omega-3 fatty acids 79–80
    polyunsaturated 81
    saturated 80
    trans fats 80
Fearnley-Whittingstall, Hugh 75
firm tofu 230

Firm Tofu with Spring Onions 154
fish 78–84
  amount eaten by the Japanese 79
  concerns over safety 82
  consumption guidelines (FSA) 83
  FSA recommendations 81–3
  health benefits 79–80, 81–2
  oily fish 81–3
  source of omega-3 fatty acids
    79–80, 81
  tips for enjoying more 84
  types of oily fish 82
fish recipes
  Alaska Salmon 155–6
  Body and Soul Warming Soba
    Buckwheat Noodles with
    Sardine & Spinach 209–10
  Dashi – Japanese Fish Cooking
    Stock 168–9
  Grilled Mackerel 199
  Grilled Salmon, Broccoli &
    Onions over Fluffy Rice 200–1
  Salmon Chahan (Fried Rice)
    173–4
  Sardines & Cherry Tomatoes
    198
  Scrambled Tofu with Salmon 201
  Seafood Medley over Sushi Rice
    178–9
  Simmered Bass in Mild Teriyaki
    Sauce 190–9
  White Fish, Firm Tofu, Leeks,
    Carrots, String Beans in Hearty
    One Pot Dish with Lime Juice
    202–3
Fisher, M. F. K. 99
Flipse, Robyn 125
Fluffy Japanese Short- or Medium-
    grain Rice (brown, white or
    haiga) 97–8
food journal 42
  sample sheet 44
food labelling 140–4
  traffic light scheme 151
food shopping guide 113–18
  farmers' markets 115–16
  food lists 114–15, 116–18
  Japanese food markets 116–17
  supermarket ready meals 138–51

supermarket shopping 113–15
  time-saving short cuts 117–18
Fox, Dr Peter 53
fruit
  Hand to Mouth – Ready to Eat
    Fruits: Strawberries, Cherries,
    Plums, Grapes, Bananas 215
  Sliced Fuji Apples with Cheeses
    214–15
  Sliced Seasonal Fruits: Apples,
    Mangoes, Watermelons,
    Melons, Pears, Peaches, Plums
    215
  Very Berries: Strawberries,
    Blueberries & Raspberries 215
  see also vegetables and fruits
FSA (Food Standards Agency) 3, 4,
    14, 20, 21, 102
  fruit and vegetable requirements
    69
  healthy beverages 109–10
  recommendations on fish 81–3

Gardner, Christopher 18, 73–4
genetics, and Japanese healthy life
    expectancy 27–8
Genmaicha green tea 109, 219
  how to brew 111–12
Genmaimacha green tea 219
  how to brew 111–12
green teas 108–9, 219–20
  health claims 108
  how to brew 111–12
  types of 109
Grilled Mackerel 199
Grilled Portabello Mushroom Open
    Sandwich with Creamy Tofu
    Sauce 191–2
Grilled Salmon, Broccoli & Onions
    over Fluffy Rice 200–1
Gyokuro green tea 219
  how to brew 111

Hand to Mouth – Ready to Eat
    Fruits: Strawberries, Cherries,
    Plums, Grapes, Bananas 215
'Harvard Healthy Eating Plan' 20
Haslam, Dr David 106
Hawks, Professor Steven R. 54

'Healthwise Plan' eating plan 20
healthy eating 4–5
   and calories 23
   eight top tips 21
   scientific evidence 22
healthy eating plans, consensus
   among 20–3
healthy life expectancy
   comparison of countries 26–7
   Japan 25–6
Hearn, Lafcadio 153
heart disease risk, and soya 89
Heart UK 102
Heller, Samantha 23
high-calorie-dense foods 68
Hill, Dr James 53, 58, 122
Hill, Professor Jim 125
hiyamugi (white flour) noodles 222
Hojicha green tea 109, 219
   how to brew 111–12
Holy Grail of Diets 20–3
Hu, Dr Frank 18, 25
Hutton, Dame Deirdre 14, 16
hypertension 15

Ishige, Naomichi 99–101

Japan Diet
   12 basic steps 1–2
   attitude 32–3
   healthy goals 38–42, 43
   natural attitude 158–60
   philosophy 3
   pre-start self-assessment 40–2
   preparation for 37–42
   recipes 166–216
   sample breakfasts 161–2
   sample dinners 163–4
   sample lunches 162–3
   sample meals based on recipes
      161–5
   sample snacks 164–5
   sharing with family and friends 37
Japan Diet away from home 131–6
   for the office 136
   in restaurants 132–5
   on-the-go snacks 135
   portion sizes in restaurants 135
   research in advance 132

when travelling 136
Japan Diet sample 7-day healthy
   eating plan 137–51
   7-day convenient healthy eating
      plan 146–51
   availability of some Japan-style
      staples 145
   home cooking 137–8
   supermarket ready meals 138–51
Japanese Country Style Simmered
   Chicken, Broccoli & Carrot
   204–5
Japanese diet 24–5
   comparison with UK diet 29–31
   levels of salt/sodium 34–5
Japanese food
   mindful eating 50–3
   popularity in the UK 45–6
Japanese food markets 116–17
Japanese people
   cancer incidence 28
   effects of Western diet 27–8
   genetic effects on health 27–8
   healthy life expectancy 25–6
   life expectancy 25–6
   link between diet and health
      25–8
   migrant studies 27–8
   obesity rates 25
Japanese teas 219–20
   Genmaicha 111–12, 109, 219
   Genmaimacha 111–12, 219
   Gyokuro 219
   Hojicha 109, 111–12, 219
   Mugicha (barley tea) 109, 112,
      219
   Sencha 109, 111, 219
   Shin-cha 219
   tea leaves, tea bags and bottles 220
Japanese Vegetarian (Shiitake
   Mushroom) Cooking Stock 167
Japanised Western meal layout 59
Japan-style eating 4–5, 7
   meal layout 60
   portion control 60–63
   quick and easy dinner menu
      154–8
   stir-fried vegetables 74–5
Jebb, Dr Susan A. 58–9

Kinpira Carrots with Hot Chilli
    Peppers 192–3
Kirby, Jane 3
kishimen (white flour) noodles 222
kombu seaweed 77, 225
Kuller, Dr Lewis 27–8, 78–80

Lansley, Andrew 15
Lambert-Lagacé, Louise 61
Lean, Professor Mike 48–9
life expectancy see healthy life
    expectancy
Lightly Sautéed Five Colour Veggies
    & Tofu Chunks 190–1
low-calorie-dense foods 68
low-carb diets 18
Lowden, Jacqui 47
Ludwig, Dr David 5
lunch, sample meals based on
    recipes 162–3

MacAvilly, Clare 42
Manson, Dr JoAnn 127
Marks & Spencer 'Eat Well' range 151
Marks & Spencer 'Healthily
    Balanced' range 151
Marting, Dr Robert N. 21, 40
Matsuri Japanese restaurant, London
    47
Mayer Stinchecum, Amanda 92
meat
    Beef, Sweet Potato and Onion
        Casserole – one pot dish 206–7
    Chicken & Eggs (Parent & Child)
        over Fluffy Rice 205–6
    Japanese Country Style Simmered
        Chicken, Broccoli & Carrot
        204–5
Mediterranean Diet 34, 73
mindful eating 50–3
mindful shopping and dining tips
    55–6
mirin (cooking wine) 220
miso (fermented soya paste) 220–1
    low-sodium options 36
Miso Soup with Baby Spinach
    156–7
Miso Soup with Clams & Mitsuba
    182

Miso Soup with Extra Firm Tofu &
    Spring Onions 181
Miso Soup with Wakame Sea
    Vegetable & Spring Onions
    183
mitsuba (Japanese parsley, trefoil)
    221
monounsaturated fats 81
Moore, Cindy 40
Morrisons 'Eat Smart' range 151
Mugicha (cold barley tea) 109, 219
    how to brew 112
mushrooms
    Grilled Portabello Mushroom
        Open Sandwich with Creamy
        Tofu Sauce 191–2
    Soba Buckwheat Noodles with
        Shiitake, Crimini Mushrooms
        & Garlic Sauce 211
    Vegetable Gyoza Dumplings
        194–6

Naomi's quick and easy Japan-style
    dinner menu 154–7
Nestle, Professor Marion 58, 88
nira (Chinese chives or garlic
    chives) 221
'No Fad Diet' 20
noodles 221–3 see also soba noodles
nori (seaweed) 77, 225

obesity
    and premature death 14
    associated health problems
        14–15
    causes of 16–19
    childhood obesity and TV
        viewing 106
    difficulties of doing research
        17–19
    lack of knowledge about 17–19
    many factors involved 18–19
    WHO definition 41
    world-wide problem 15
obesity levels
    among children 14–15
    in the UK 14–15
    Japan 14, 15
    USA 14, 15

oils
  rapeseed/canola oil 101–2, 223
  sesame oil 223–4
oily fish *see* fish
Oliver, Jamie 107
omega-3 fatty acids
  from fish 79–80, 81
  in the Japanese diet 79
organic fruit and vegetables 70

panko (Japanese breadcrumbs) 224
passive overeating 58
Phillips, Dr Frankie 17, 32, 69,
  138–51
phytochemicals 68–9
plate size in Japan 58, 59
polyunsaturated fats 81
portable Japan Diet 131–6
portion control
  Bento Box 62–3
  Japan-style 60–63
portion size
  and excess calories 57–8
  in Japan 58–9
  on the increase 57–8
  passive overeating 58

Radish Salad 184–5
rapeseed/canola oil 101–2, 223
recipes for the Japan Diet 166–216
  cooking stocks 167–9
  dressings, sauces & marinades
    170–2
  fish dishes 198–203
  meat dishes 204–7
  rice dishes 173–9
  salads 184–8
  snacks 214–16
  soba noodle dishes 208–13
  soups 180–3
  vegetable dishes 189–97
Renton, Alex 46
rice 91–8
  electric rice cooker 96–7, 98
  Glycemic Index of white rice
    94–5
  health benefits 92–3
  Japanese-style short-grain rice
    93–6, 218

non-stick rice paddle (shamoji)
  232
  variety of uses 91–2
  ways to eat more 96–7
  white rice and weight gain 94–5
rice recipes
  Brown Rice 156
  Fluffy Japanese Short- or
    Medium-grain Rice (brown,
    white or haiga) 97–8
  Rice with Edamame Soya Beans
    173
  Salmon Chahan (Fried Rice)
    173–4
  Seafood Medley over Sushi Rice
    178–9
  Tri-colour Vegetables over Sushi
    Rice 176–7
  Vinegared Sushi Rice 175–6
rice vinegar 224
rice wine (sake) 224–5
Rice with Edamame Soya Beans 173
Rolls, Dr Barbara 68, 87

Sainsbury's 'Be Good to Yourself'
  range 140–1, 146–50
Sakata, Dr Toshiie 53
salads
  Asparagus Salad with White
    Sesame Dressing 184
  Beetroot Leaves Salad with Lemon
    Dressing 187
  Chilled Cucumber Salad 185
  Cool Summer Soba Buckwheat
    Noodle Salad 208–9
  Edamame Mesclun Salad 186
  Radish Salad 184–5
  Seared Jumbo Prawns on a bed of
    Mesclun Salad 188
  Summer Ripe Tomato & Tofu
    Salad 185–6
Salmon Chahan (Fried Rice) 173–4
salt content
  proposed labelling 151
  supermarket healthy meals 142–3
salt in the diet 34–6
  recommended amounts 35
  sources 35–6
  tips to reduce 35–6

Sardines & Cherry Tomatoes 198
Sass, Cynthia 75
saturated fats 80
sauces
  Creamy Tofu Sauce 171
  dipping sauce for Vegetable
    Gyoza Dumplings 195
Sautéed Beetroots 189
Schwarcz, Professor Joe 79
Schwartz, Dr Lisa 17
Scrambled Tofu with Salmon 201
sea vegetables (seaweed) 76–7,
  225–6
  health benefits 77
  kombu 225
  nori 225–6
  sushi nori 226
  wakame 226
seafood
  Miso Soup with Clams & Mitsuba
    182
  Seafood Medley over Sushi Rice
    178–9
  Seared Jumbo Prawns on a bed of
    Mesclun Salad 188
Sencha green tea 109, 219
  how to brew 111
sesame oil 223–4
Sesame Oil Salad Dressing 170
sesame seeds (goma) 226–7
shichimi togarashi (seven-spice mix)
    227
Shin-cha 219
shiso (herb) 227
Sikora, Professor Karol 19, 28
silken tofu 229–30
Simmered Bass in Mild Teriyaki
    Sauce 198–9
Simmered Daikon & Tofu 196–7
Simmered Mixed Vegetables 155
Simon, Dr Harvey 123
Simons-Morton, Dr Denise 130
Skibola, Dr Christine 77
Sliced Fuji Apples with Cheeses
    214–15
Sliced Seasonal Fruits: Apples,
  Mangoes, Watermelons,
  Melons, Pears, Peaches, Plums
    215

snacks
  Bananas on Toasted Multi-grain
    Bread 214
  Hand to Mouth – Ready to Eat
    Fruits: Strawberries, Cherries,
    Plums, Grapes, Bananas 215
  sample snacks based on recipes
    164–5
  Sliced Fuji Apples with Cheeses
    214–15
  Sliced Seasonal Fruits: Apples,
    Mangoes, Watermelons,
    Melons, Pears, Peaches, Plums
    215
  Steamed Sweet Potatoes 216
  Very Berries: Strawberries,
    Blueberries & Raspberries 215
soba (buckwheat) noodles 222
  Body and Soul Warming Soba
    Buckwheat Noodles with
    Sardine & Spinach 209–10
  Cool Summer Soba Buckwheat
    Noodle Salad 208–9
  Soba Buckwheat Noodles with
    Sautéed Green Peppers &
    String Beans with Garlic Soy
    Sauce 212–13
  Soba Buckwheat Noodles with
    Shiitake, Crimini Mushrooms
    & Garlic Sauce 211
sodium content
  proposed salt content labelling 151
  supermarket healthy meals 142–3
sodium in the diet 34–6
  recommended amounts 35
  sources 35–6
  tips to reduce 35–6
somen (white flour) noodles 222
Somerfield 'Good Intentions' range
    151
soups
  Cauliflower–Napa Cabbage 'East-
    Meets-West' Soup 180
  Miso Soup with Baby Spinach
    156–7
  Miso Soup with Clams & Mitsuba
    182
  Miso Soup with Extra Firm Tofu
    & Spring Onions 181

Miso Soup with Wakame Sea
    Vegetable & Spring Onions
    183
soy sauce (shoyu), reduced-sodium
    type 36, 227–8
soya 85–90
    and breast cancer risk 88–9
    and heart disease risk 89
    edamame 87
    health claims for 88–9
    in the Japanese diet 86
    protein source 86–7
    ways to include in your diet 90
soya beans (edamame) 87
    Edamame Mesclun Salad 186
    Rice with Edamame Soya Beans
        173
Stampfer, Dr Meir 15
Steamed Sweet Potatoes 216
Steamed Veggies with Ginger Soy
    Sauce 189–90
steaming food 102–4
Steffen, Dr Lyn 69
stir-fried vegetables, Japan-style
    74–5
sugar consumption
    Japan 106–7
    sweetened fizzy drinks 105–6
    UK 107
Summer Ripe Tomato & Tofu Salad
    185–6
superfoods formula 64
supermarket shopping 113–15
    availability of some Japan-style
        staples 145
    healthy ready meal choices
        138–51
    sales of Japanese foods 46
sushi
    nutritional benefits 48–9
    seaweed wrapping 77
    wooden sushi tub (hangiri sushi
        oke) 232
sushi lunch, benefits of 46–7
sushi nori 226
sushi recipes, Vinegared Sushi Rice
    175–6
sushi shops, popularity in the UK
    45–6

Sutton, Louise 126
sweet potato 75–6
    Beef, Sweet Potato and Onion
        Casserole – one pot dish 206–7
    Steamed Sweet Potatoes 216
sweetened fizzy drinks, health
    effects 105–7

tamari 228–9
tea leaves, tea bags and bottles 220
teas see green teas; Japanese teas
teriyaki sauce, low-sodium options
    36
Tesco 'Healthy Living' range 141–2,
    146–50
'Therapeutic Lifestyle Changes'
    (TLC) eating plan 20
Till, Dr Simon 123–4
Toasted & Ground White Sesame
    Seeds 171
tofu 85–7, 228–30
    firm tofu 230
    silken tofu 229–30
    yakidofu tofu 230
tofu recipes
    Cool Summer Soba Buckwheat
        Noodle Salad 208–9
    Creamy Tofu Sauce 171
    Firm Tofu with Spring Onions
        154
    Grilled Portabello Mushroom
        Open Sandwich with Creamy
        Tofu Sauce 191–2
    Lightly Sautéed Five Colour
        Veggies & Tofu Chunks 190–1
    Miso Soup with Extra Firm Tofu
        & Spring Onions 181
    Scrambled Tofu with Salmon 201
    Simmered Daikon & Tofu 196–7
    Summer Ripe Tomato & Tofu
        Salad 185–6
    White Fish, Firm Tofu, Leeks,
        Carrots, String Beans in Hearty
        One Pot Dish with Lime Juice
        202–3
Tokyo, food choices 11
Tokyo kitchen key ingredients
    217–32
    bonito (fish) flakes (katsuo-bushi,

hana-katsuo or kezuribushi) 217
daikon (large white radish) 217–8
edamame (fresh green soya beans) 218
firm tofu 230
Genmaicha 219
Genmaimacha 219
green teas 219
Gyokuro 219
hiyamugi (white flour) noodles 222
Hojicha 219
Japanese-style short-grain rice 218
Japanese teas 219–20
kishimen (white flour) noodles 222
kombu 225
mirin (cooking wine) 220
miso (fermented soya paste) 220–1
mitsuba (Japanese parsley, trefoil) 221
Mugicha (barley tea) 219–20
nira (Chinese chives or garlic chives) 221
noodles 221–3
nori 225–6
oils 223–4
panko (Japanese breadcrumbs) 224
rapeseed/canola oil 223
rice vinegar 224
rice wine (sake) 224–5
sea vegetables (seaweed) 225–6
Sencha 219
sesame oil 223–4
sesame seeds (goma) 226
shichimi togarashi (seven-spice mix) 227
Shin-cha 219
shiso (herb) 227
silken tofu 229–30
soba (buckwheat) noodles 222
somen (white flour) noodles 222
soy sauce (shoyu), reduced-sodium type 227–8
tamari 228
tea leaves, tea bags and bottles 220

tofu 228–30
udon (white flour) noodles 222–3
wakame 226
wasabi 231
yakidofu tofu 230
yuzu (Citrus junos) 231
Tokyo kitchen utensils
drop-lid (otoshi buta) 232
non-stick rice paddle (shamoji) 232
wooden sushi tub (hangiri sushi oke) 232
tomatoes
Sardines & Cherry Tomatoes 198
Summer Ripe Tomato & Tofu Salad 185–6
Traditional Japanese Vinaigrette 170
trans fats 80
Tri-colour Vegetables over Sushi Rice 176–7
Turner, Brian 75

udon (white flour) noodles 222–3
UK, healthy life expectancy 27
UK diet
comparison with Japanese diet 29–31
salt/sodium levels 34–5
UK Heart Foundation 22
US, healthy life expectancy 27
US National Institutes for Health 22, 23

Valignano, Alessandro 45
vegetable recipes
Aubergine & Green Peppers with Red Miso Dressing 193–4
Grilled Portabello Mushroom Open Sandwich with Creamy Tofu Sauce 191–2
Kinpira Carrots with Hot Chilli Peppers 192–3
Lightly Sautéed Five Colour Veggies & Tofu Chunks 190–1
Sautéed Beetroots 189
Simmered Daikon & Tofu 196–7
Simmered Mixed Vegetables 155

Soba Buckwheat Noodles with
  Sautéed Green Peppers &
  String Beans with Garlic Soy
  Sauce 212–13
Steamed Veggies with Ginger Soy
  Sauce 189–90
Tri-colour Vegetables over Sushi
  Rice 176–7
Vegetable Gyoza Dumplings
  194–6
White Fish, Firm Tofu, Leeks,
  Carrots, String Beans in Hearty
  One Pot Dish with Lime Juice
  202–3
vegetables
  nutritional benefits 73–4
  sample menu of vegetable dishes
    66
  sea vegetables (seaweed) 76
  sweet potato 75–6
vegetables and fruits 64–72
  beneficial substances 68–9
  help in weight loss 68
  organic 70
  recommended intake 69–70
  ways to increase your intake 71–2
Very Berries: Strawberries,
  Blueberries & Raspberries 215
Vinegared Sushi Rice 175–6
Vogel, Professor Robert 34

waist measurement
  and health risks 41–2
  measure of fat level 41–2
Waitrose 'Perfectly Balanced' range
  140, 146–50
wakame (seaweed) 77, 226
walking, health benefits 127
wasabi 231
Weeden, Paul 76
weight gain

and speed of eating 53–4
and Western diet 6–7
weight loss 4
  and calories 23
  and eating slowly 53–4
  preparation for 37–42
  with Japan-style eating 7–10
weight loss maintenance, and
  exercise 125
'Weight Watchers' 20
Western diet and weight gain 6–7
White Fish, Firm Tofu, Leeks,
  Carrots, String Beans in Hearty
  One Pot Dish with Lime Juice
  202–3
white rice see rice
White Sesame Seed Dressing 172
WHO (World Health Organization)
  3, 22, 25
  fish consumption 81
  sweetened fizzy drinks and
    obesity 106
  TV viewing and childhood
    obesity 106
wholegrains 91–8
  health benefits 92–3
  ways to eat more 96–7
  wholegrain foods 93
Whyte, Dr John J. 21, 40
Willett, Dr Walter 18, 82, 94
Wing, Dr Rena 122
Woloshin, Dr Steven 17
Worrall Thompson, Antony 75

yakidofu tofu 230
Yanovski, Dr Susan 17
Yelmokas McDermott, Dr Ann 31,
  53, 65, 125
Yong, Ed 67, 88
yuba 85
yuzu (Citrus junos) 231

JAPANESE WOMEN DON'T GET OLD OR FAT

'I take a deep breath.

I am in my mother's Tokyo kitchen.

I am drenched in a narcotic mixture of subtle, sweet and earthy fragrances I've tasted since I was a little girl.

The kitchen smells like the earth, the sea and the mountains . . . it smells like life.'

There is a land where women live longer than everyone else on Earth.

It is a place where obesity is the lowest in the developed world.

Where forty-year-old women look like they are twenty.

It is a land where women enjoy some of the world's most delicious food, yet they have obesity rates of only 3 per cent – less than one-third that of French women . . . and less than one-tenth that of American women.

It is a country of women obsessed with enjoying life – and mastering the art of healthy eating. It is a highly industrialised nation that is the second-largest economic power in the world.

The country is Japan.

And something incredible is happening there.

Filled with evocative reminiscences of a childhood spent in Tokyo, *Japanese Women Don't Get Old or Fat* shows that Japanese ingredients are not about complicated sushi or elaborate formal dining, but about everyday cooking that has stood the test of time – and waistlines – for decades.

The perfect accompaniment to *The Japan Diet*!

About the Authors

Naomi Moriyama is the bestselling author of *Japanese Women Don't Get Old or Fat*. She was born and raised in Tokyo and spent childhood summers on her grandparents' hillside farm in the Japanese countryside. Naomi attended college in Illinois, where she gained 25 pounds eating pizza and biscuits before moving back to Japan and re-discovering the secrets of her mother Chizuko's Tokyo kitchen.

Naomi lives in Manhattan with her husband and co-author, William Doyle, and travels to her mother's Tokyo kitchen several times a year.

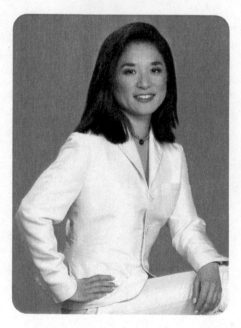

William Doyle is an award-winning writer and co-author of the bestselling *Japanese Women Don't Get Old or Fat*. He was born in New York and has travelled widely in Japan.